Freestyle Slow Cooker Recipes

All New Delicious Freestyle 2018 Recipes For Busy Person Weight Loss goals with minimal effort

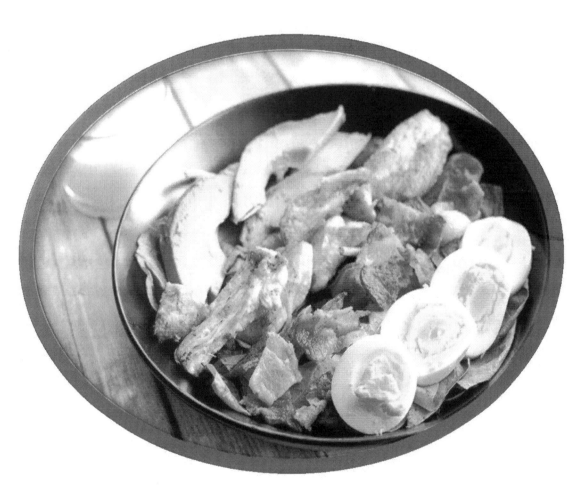

By P Simon

Before you embark on the journey to learning how to follow the ketogenic diet to bring about different benefits, it is best that you have a good understanding of what the diet is about. This knowledge will help you to approach the diet from a point of knowledge, as opposed to just preparing recipes that you don't understand why they are there in the first place. This knowledge will also help you to customize your own recipes easily.

Table of Contents

Introduction

I want to thank you and congratulate you for buying my book

This book has actionable information about the Weight Watchers diet, and Slow Cooking including 120 delicious Weight Watchers Freestyle 2018 slow cooker recipes that you can prepare to get started.

And this book will show you exactly what you need to do to move from where you are i.e. unhealthy, overweight/obese, to where you want to be i.e. of healthy weight and with good overall health.

In this book, you will learn what the Weight Watchers and its new Freestyle diet is all about including what it is you should eat, what you should not eat, how it works, why it works, the benefits that come with following a ketogenic diet, 120 delicious recipes that you can prepare fast and much, much more.

Let's begin!

Thanks again for getting this book. I hope you enjoy it!

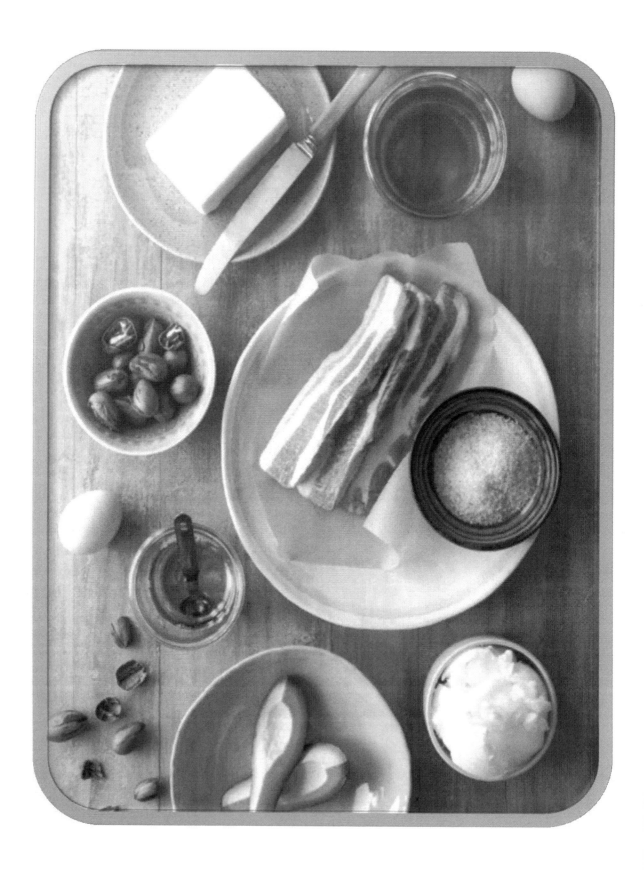

What Is Slow Cooking?

Slow cookers are not new appliances in the culinary world. They have been around for decades; you might even have fond memories from your childhood of your parents serving your favorite dinner out of one. Slow cookers are very versatile because the cooking environment works the same no matter the cuisine. Knowing what slow cookers can and can't do is important for planning your meals, especially for a diet like keto.

In this chapter, you will learn slow-cooker basics such as which kind is best for your needs, how to ensure your recipes turn out great, and how to convert your traditional family favorites to work for you. Taking the mystery out of the slow cooker should give you the confidence to create spectacular meals as often as you want in order to reach your goals while eating well.

Why Cook Slow?

You might be wondering why you should invest in a slow cooker when other cooking techniques produce perfectly fine meals. Some of the reasons to use a slow cooker include:

Enhances flavor: Cooking ingredients over several hours with spices, herbs, and other seasonings creates vegetables and proteins that burst with delicious flavors. This slow process allows the flavors to mellow and deepen for an enhanced eating experience.

Saves time: Cooking at home takes a great deal of time: prepping, sautéing, stirring, turning the heat up and down, and watching the meal so that it does not over- or undercook. If you're unable to invest the time, you might find yourself reaching for convenience foods instead of healthy choices. Slow cookers allow you to do other activities while the meal cooks. You can put your ingredients in the slow cooker in the morning and come home to a perfectly cooked meal.

Convenient: Besides the time-saving aspect, using a slow cooker can free up the stove and oven for other dishes. This can be very convenient for large holiday meals or when you want to serve a side dish and entrée as well as a delectable dessert. Clean up is simple when you use the slow cooker for messy meals because most inserts are nonstick or are easily cleaned with a little soapy water, and each meal is prepared in either just the machine or using one additional vessel to sauté ingredients. There is no wide assortment of pots, pans, and baking dishes to contend with at the end of the day.

Low heat production: If you have ever cooked dinner on a scorching summer afternoon, you will appreciate the low amount of heat produced by a slow cooker. Even after eight hours of operation, slow cookers do not heat up your kitchen and you will not be sweating over the hot stovetop. Slow cookers use about a third of the energy of conventional cooking methods, just a little more energy than a traditional light bulb.

Supports healthy eating: Cooking your food at high heat can reduce the nutrition profile of your foods, breaking down and removing the majority of vitamins, minerals, and antioxidants while producing unhealthy chemical compounds that can contribute to disease. Low-heat cooking retains all the goodness that you want for your diet.

Saves Money: Slow cookers save you money because of the low amount of electricity they use and because the best ingredients for slow cooking are the less expensive cuts of beef and heartier inexpensive vegetables. Tougher cuts of meat—brisket, chuck, shanks—break down beautifully to fork-tender goodness. Another cost-saving benefit is that most 6-quart slow cookers will produce enough of a recipe to stretch your meals over at least two days. Leftovers are one of the best methods for saving money.

Slow Cooker or Crock Pot?

Slow cooker is the generic name for an appliance that has heating elements all around the insert that quickly bring food up to safe temperatures. In 1971, the Rival Company released its own slow-cooker product to the market, which it called the Crock-Pot. Just as many people refer to tissues as Kleenex, often people use the words slow cooker and Crock-Pot interchangeably. But while all Crock-Pots are slow cookers, not all slow cookers are Crock-Pots. Other popular slow-cooker brands include All-Clad, Cuisinart, and Hamilton Beach.

Slow Cooking Methods

There are two methods for cooking food: moist or dry heat. Ovens, grills, and panfrying use dry heat. Moist-heat methods include braising, stewing, and steaming. Slow cookers fall in the moist-heat category because of their low-temperature, closed-cooking environment. This method is perfect for tough cuts of meat and breaking down fibrous vegetables. Temperature and steam both come into play to create this favorable environment.

Temperature

Slow cookers feature a range of temperatures for convenience. Basic slow cookers have low and high settings, and more advanced models include digital displays for exact temperatures and probes that can be inserted. The recipes in this book are geared toward low-heat cooking, about 180°F to 200°F, so that any liquid simmers gently at a food-safe 185°F and the timing is long. The best temperature to create tender meats is 180°F; it is high enough for connective tissues to break down into tenderizing gelatin but low enough that the meat will not overcook. Low settings also allow you to assemble your recipe and then leave the house for a regular workday while it cooks without compromising food quality or health.

High settings cook recipes approximately twice as fast. As a result, high-heat recipes can require some supervision to avoid overcooking meats or more delicate ingredients. Also, if you cook your food too fast, it might sit longer before you eat it, which is not safe. Two hours is the maximum time any recipe should be held on the "warm" setting. If you are planning to be home or need your meal quicker, then high heat in a slow cooker works fine for most recipes besides desserts and those that require baking.

Steam

Slow cookers have a tight-fitting lid that traps the steam created as the food cooks and the temperature heats up in the insert. The liquid in the slow cooker simmers creating steam, which very gently cooks the ingredients without compromising flavor and texture. As this steam is produced, this locked environment inhibits bacteria growth, so lifting the lid during the cooking process can be done once or twice to check progress, but multiple times is not recommended. The steamy environment is limiting because it does not allow meats to brown, vegetables to caramelize, and the skin of poultry to crisp up. All of these effects require dry heat. So there are some recipes that aren't best for your slow cooker.

Slow Cooking Myths

Slow cookers have been around for a long time, and most people have tried them at one point or another, sometimes successfully and other times not. When the results aren't perfect, false assumptions crop up. Some of the most common myths surrounding slow cookers are:

You can't open the lid. This is a recommendation, but you can open the lid without ruining your meal. Lifting the lid will drop the temperature 15 to 30°F depending on how long the lid is off the insert. If done early in the timing, 2 to 3 hours in a 6-hour recipe, then you should extend the time 30 minutes. If you lift the lid near the end, it won't affect anything at all.

All the recipes taste the same. Any type of cuisine, from South American to Indian, can be made in a slow cooker. Spices and flavors deepen in the slow cooker, so your meals should be more flavorful than standard cooking methods no matter what kind of food you are cooking. If your recipes all taste the same, you might be using similar recipes or seasonings.

You have to completely fill the insert. Many slow cooker recipes produce a vast amount of food because the insert is filled completely. You don't have to do this. Filling the insert halfway or one-third of the way simply means adjusting the time to fewer hours. The more food in the insert, the more time on the timer.

You have to precook ingredients. Precooking can be beneficial for certain types of ingredients, such as red meats and poultry with skin. However, you do not have to precook any of your ingredients at all. Browned meat and chicken are more attractive and have a richer flavor than meat that hasn't been browned, but there isn't a vast difference between the two. You will still enjoy a delicious meal if you skip this step. It's a good idea to remove poultry skin though, because the texture is a little unpleasant without time in the skillet.

You're limited to stews and casseroles. Slow cookers are incredibly versatile, and recipes have come a long way over the decades. Desserts, breads, side dishes, glazed meats, and even granola can be made effectively in a slow cooker with fabulous results. Soups, stews, chili, and braised meats are still slow-cooker staples because they turn out particularly well, but you can make almost anything—and make it delicious.

Do More with Crock Pot

Slow cookers are wonderful for many types of dishes, but they certainly cannot be used for everything you will eat on the diet. Obviously, grilled and broiled meats are impossible because delicious caramelization is not possible with a slow cooker. This is why precooking is recommended for some meats and poultry. You can bake in the slow cooker, but the browning that occurs in dry heat will not happen. As stated elsewhere in this book, recipes that incorporate dairy products from the beginning of a recipe do not turn out well. The long cooking times in slow cookers causes dairy to split, and you end up with lumps of whey bound to casein. Here are some foods and dishes that are not ideally suited for slow cookers:

Tender cuts of meat such as beef sirloin or beef tenderloin

Seafood

Delicate vegetables such as asparagus or lettuces (unless added at the very end)

Fresh herbs (unless added at the very end)

Dairy products (unless added at the very end)

Choosing Your Crock Pot

Slow cookers have changed a lot over the years. These days you can purchase models that range from very simple models all the way to ones that look like they should be on a space station. When buying the right model for your needs, you have to consider what you are cooking, how many portions, and if you will be home during the cooking process. All these factors are important when deciding on the size, shape, and features of your slow cooker.

Size and Shape

Slow cookers come in a multitude of sizes and shapes, so it is important to consider your needs and what will work best for the type of food prepared on the keto diet. There are models that range from ½-quart to large 8-quart models and everything in-between.

The small slow cookers (½-quart to 2-quart) are usually used for dips or sauces, as well as recipes designed for one person. Medium-sized slow cookers (3-quart to 4-quart) are great for baking or for meals that create food for two to three people. The slow cooker recommended for most of the recipes in this book is the 5-quart to 6-quart model because it is perfect for the large cuts of meat on the diet and can prepare food for four people, including leftovers. The enormous 7-quart to 8-quart appliance is meant for very large meals. If you have money in your budget, owning both a 3-quart and 6-quart model would be the best of both worlds.

When it comes to shapes, you will have to decide between round, oval, and rectangular. Round slow cookers are fine for stews and chili, but do not work well for large pieces of meat. These should probably not be your choice. Oval and rectangular slow cookers both allow for the ingredients you will use regularly that are large, like roasts, ribs, and chops, and have the added advantage of fitting loaf pans, ramekins, and casserole dishes, as well. Some desserts and breads are best cooked in another container placed in the slow cooker, and you will see several recipes in this book that use that technique.

Features

Now that you know the size and shape of the recommended slow cooker, it is time to consider what you want this appliance to do for you. Depending on your budget, at a minimum you want a slow cooker with temperature controls that cover warm, low, and high, as well as a removable insert. These are the primary features of the bare-bones models that will get the job done. However, if you want to truly experience a set-it-and-forget-it appliance that creates the best meals possible in this cooking environment, you might want to consider the following features:

Digital programmable controls: You can program temperature, when the slow cooker starts, how long it cooks, and when the slow cooker switches to warm.

Glass lid: These are heavier, and allow you to look into the slow cooker without removing them, so there is little heat loss. Opt for a lid with clamps, and you can transport your cooked meal easily to parties and gatherings if needed.

Temperature probe: Once you have a slow cooker with this feature, you will wonder how you cooked previously without it. The temperature probe allows you to cook your meat, poultry, and egg dishes to an exact temperature and then switches to warm when completed.

Precooking feature: Some models have a precooking feature that allows you to brown your meat and poultry right in the insert. You will still have to take the time to do this step, but you won't have a skillet to clean afterward.

IF YOU DON'T HAVE A PROGRAMMABLE SLOW COOKER

If you opt for a basic, analog slow cooker—the kind with a dial—or already have one that is not programmable, there is still an option if you want to control the cooking time. This might be something to consider if you are usually away from your home more than the time needed for the recipes you are cooking. A socket timer—the same kind that people use to switch their lights on and off when on vacation—is a great hack to turn your basic slow cooker into a programmable model. You simply plug your slow cooker into it, turn your slow cooker to the desired high or low setting, and set the timer for how long the cooking process should take, and when you want it to turn on or off. This timer will only work if you have a slow cooker that is set with a dial because a digital model needs to be manually set when turned on. For food-safety reasons, the ingredients need to be completely chilled in the insert until you are ready to leave the house and the timer should not be set for prolonged periods of time.

Tips for Slow Cooking

Slow cookers are simple to use, but you can increase your success with a few tips and techniques. In the following list, some tips are suggestions and some should be considered more seriously for safety or health reasons. The intent is to provide the best information possible so that your meals are delicious and easy.

Always

1. **Read the user manual and any other literature.** You will find an assortment of instructions included in the slow-cooker box so take the time to sit down and read everything completely before using a new device. You might think you know how everything works, but each model is a little different and it is best to be informed about all of the things your slow cooker can do.

2. **Grease the insert of the slow cooker before cooking.** Cleaning a slow cooker insert can be a challenge, so grease the insert, even for soups and stews. You don't want to scrub the insert with abrasive brushes or scraping bits of cooked-on food off, because you will wreck its nonstick surface.

3. **Add dairy and herbs at the end of the cooking process.** As stated elsewhere in this book, dairy and fresh herbs do not hold up well during long cooking times. Dairy splits and creates a grainy, unpleasant texture, and herbs lose their flavor, color, and texture. Always add these ingredients at the end.

4. **Always cut your ingredients into similar-sized pieces.** Slow cookers are not meant to be used for staggered cooking recipes such as stir-fries where the more delicate ingredients are added last to avoid overcooking. Evenly sized pieces mean your ingredients will be ready at the same time and your meals will be cooked evenly.

5. **Adjust your seasonings.** Slow cookers can have an unexpected effect on herbs and spices so it is important to taste and adjust at the end of the process. Some spices, such as curry or cayenne, can get more intense, while the long cooking time can reduce the impact of dried herbs. It is best to hold off on too much salt until the very end as well because it will get stronger.

Never

1. **Add too much liquid.** Very little evaporation occurs in a slow cooker compared to stovetop or oven cooking. Most slow cooker recipes, with the exception of soups and sauces, call for 50 percent less liquid than conventional ones.

2. **Use frozen meats or poultry.** The ingredients in slow cookers need to reach 140°F within 4 hours for food safety, so large cuts of meat or poultry should be fully thawed. You can add small frozen items like meatballs to a slow cooker because these can come to temperature within this time range.

3. **Place your insert right from the refrigerator into the slow cooker.** When you remove your previously prepared meal from the refrigerator, let the insert sit out at room temperature for 30 minutes or so to avoid cracking it with extreme temperature changes. Also, never remove the hot insert from your slow cooker and place it on a cold surface.

4. **Resume cooking after a power outage of over two hours.** Power outages can happen in any season, and for food-safety reasons, you have to err on the side of caution. If an outage lasts for more than two hours, especially during the first few hours of the cooking time, you need to discard the food because the amount of time spent in the food danger zone (40°F to 140°F) will have been too long. If the outage is less than two hours and it occurs after your food has been cooking for at least four hours, then you can resume cooking until the end of the original time or transfer the food to a pot or casserole dish and finish it on the stove or in the oven. When in doubt, throw the food out.

5. **Use the recommended cooking times in high altitudes.** As with most other cooking methods, slow cookers need more cooking time if you live above an altitude of 3,000 feet. The liquid in the slow cooker will simmer at a lower temperature so high-heat settings are recommended, or if you can program the slow cooker, then set it to maintain the food at 200°F or higher. You can also use a temperature probe set to 165°F internal temperature if your slow cooker has this feature.

Making Your Favorite Recipes to Cook

If you have a recipe that is a tried-and-true family favorite, you might be able to convert it for your slow cooker. Obviously, if you are trying to adapt Uncle Bob's famous grilled beef tenderloin, you might be out of luck. Take a look at the type of recipe and follow a few simple guidelines to convert it to a convenient slow-cooker version. These guidelines include:

Don't try recipes that require less than 15 minutes of cooking time because the ingredients will probably not hold up well enough.

Reduce the amount of liquid in the recipe, unless you are making a soup, because the sealed environment of a slow cooker creates a steaming effect where the liquid condenses on the lid and falls back into the insert. Use about half of the recommended liquid.

If the recipe does not ask for any liquid, as is the case with roasted joints of meat or poultry, add between ¼ cup and ½ cup of water or broth.

Leave out any dairy products until the end of the cooking time, or if the product is used as the only liquid, then replace it with coconut milk.

Brown your meats and poultry so that you get the same rich flavor and gorgeous color.

Make sure to convert the recipe's cook time to work with a slow cooker: 15 minutes equals 1 to 2 hours on low, 30 minutes equals 3 to 4 hours on low, 45 minutes equals 5 to 6 hours on low, 1 hour equals 6 to 8 hours on low, and 2 hours equals 9 to 10 hours on low.

Freestyle Breakfast Recipes

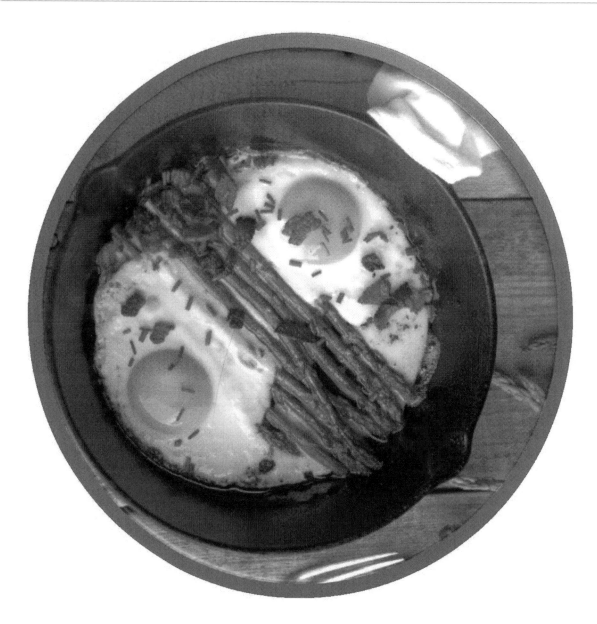

Sausage & Egg Slow Cooker Casserole

Points: 4, Serves: 6, Cooking Time: 5 hours, Preparation Time: 15 minutes

Ingredients:

- ¼ teaspoon pepper
- ½ teaspoon salt
- Cooking spray
- 2 cloves garlic minced
- ¾ cup whipping cream
- 10 eggs
- 1 cup shredded Cheddar cheese, divided
- 1 12-ounce package sausages, cooked and sliced

Instructions:

1. Grease bottom and sides of Slow Cooker with cooking spray.
2. Set to low setting.
3. In a large bowl, whisk eggs.
4. Season with pepper and salt. Mix well.
5. Stir in whipping cream and whisk to mix well.
6. In Slow Cooker, spread ½ of sliced sausages, followed by ½ of cheese, and topped by remaining sausage.
7. Pour in egg mixture and sprinkle remaining cheese on top.
8. Cover and cook for 5 hours.
9. If desired, cook on high settings for 3 hours.

Nutrition information:

Calories per serving: 496; Carbohydrates: 4.94g; Protein: 26.65g; Fat: 40.41g; Sugar: 1.85g; Sodium: 1003mg; Fiber: 0.1g

Ricotta and Spinach Egg Casserole

Points: 2, Serves: 6, Cooking Time: 7 hour, Preparation Time: 10 minutes

Ingredients:

- ¼ teaspoon salt
- Cooking spray
- 12 large eggs
- 1 cup ricotta cheese
- 9-ounce box frozen spinach, water squeezed out
- 1 small yellow onion, diced
- ¼ cup heavy whipping cream

Instructions:

1. Grease sides and bottom of Slow Cooker with cooking spray.
2. In a blender, blend until smooth the onion, ricotta cheese, whipping cream and 4 eggs.
3. Once smooth, set aside.
4. In a bowl, whisk well remaining eggs.
5. Season with salt and whisk well.

6. Stir in blended mixture and mix again.
7. Add spinach and mix well.
8. Pour into slow cooker.
9. Cover and cook on low for 7 hours or on high for 4 hours.

Nutrition information:

Calories per serving: 208; Carbohydrates: 3.19g; Protein: 10.22g; Fat: 17.02; Sugar: 0.76g; Sodium: 152mg; Fiber: 0.1g

Mustard-Zucchini Casserole

Points: 3, Serves: 6, Cooking Time: 5 hours and 30 minutes, Preparation Time: 15 minutes

Ingredients:

- Salt and Pepper to taste
- 3 large eggs
- 2 teaspoons prepared yellow mustard
- 1 ½ cheddar cheese, shredded and divided
- 2 cups diced zucchini
- 1 teaspoon dried ground sage

Instructions:

1. Grease sides and bottom of Slow Cooker with cooking spray.
2. In a bowl, whisk well eggs.
3. Season with pepper and salt.
4. Stir in ground sage and yellow mustard. Whisk well.
5. Stir in 1 cup of cheese.
6. In slow cooker spread zucchini evenly in bottom of pot.
7. Pour in egg mixture.
8. Cover and cook on low for 5 hours or on High for 3 hours.
9. Then sprinkle remaining cheese on top and cook for another 30 minutes.

Nutrition information:

Calories per serving: 147; Carbohydrates: 1.67g; Protein: 8.46g; Fat: 11.91g; Sugar: 0.53g; Sodium: 205mg; Fiber: 0.3g

Poached Salmon in Slow Cooker

Points: 3, Serves: 4, Cooking Time: hours minutes, Preparation Time: minutes

Ingredients:

- 2 cups water
- 1 teaspoon salt, and more
- 1 teaspoon black peppercorns, and more
- 2-pounds skin on salmon (4 fillets)
- 5 sprigs of dill or tarragon
- 1 bay leaf
- 1 shallot, sliced thinly
- 1 lemon, sliced thinly

Instructions:

1. In slow cooker mix salt, peppercorns, herbs, bay leaf, shallot, lemon, and lime.
2. Cover and cook for an hour on high settings.

3. Season top of salmon with pepper and salt.
4. Place in slow cooker with skin side down.
5. Cover and cook for 1.5-hours on high settings or until fish is flaky.

Nutrition information:

Calories per serving: 367; Carbohydrates: 2.13g; Protein: 59.95g; Fat: 13.35g; Sugar: 0.91g; Sodium: 1460mg; Fiber: 0.3g

Breakfast Casserole Mexican Style

Points: 4, Serves: 10, Cooking Time: 7 hours and 8 minutes, Preparation Time: minutes

Ingredients:
- ¼ teaspoon salt
- ¼ teaspoon pepper
- 12-ounces Jones Dairy Farm Pork Sausage Roll
- 10 eggs
- 1 cup cheese
- 1 cup salsa
- 1 tablespoon cilantro, chopped

Instructions:
1. Grease sides and bottom of Slow Cooker with cooking spray.
2. Set on low.
3. Place a nonstick fry pan on medium high fire and cook sausage. Breaking it into pieces as you sauté it until no longer pink, around 8 minutes. Turn off fire and transfer to slow cooker. Spread evenly on bottom of pot.
4. In a large bowl, whisk well eggs, cilantro, salt and pepper.
5. Stir in ½ cup cheese and ½ cup salsa.
6. Pour into pot.
7. Cover and cook for 6 hours. Do not open until then.
8. Once done, sprinkle cheese on top.
9. Cover and cook for an additional hour.
10. Serve with a dollop of salsa and enjoy.

Nutrition information:

Calories per serving: 297; Carbohydrates: 3.45g; Protein: 18.93g; Fat: 22.95g; Sugar: 2.17g; Sodium: 700mg; Fiber: 0.5g

Cabbage Rolls in Slow Cooker

Points: 2, Serves: 6, Cooking Time: hours minutes, Preparation Time: minutes

Ingredients:
- ½ teaspoon pepper
- ½ teaspoon salt
- 12 large cabbage leaves
- 1-pound ground beef
- 1 cup no sugar added marinara sauce
- 1 teaspoon garlic powder
- 1 teaspoon onion powder

Instructions:

1. Wrap cabbage leaves in wet paper towel and place on microwave safe plate. Microwave for 5 minutes or until leaves are slightly soft. This makes it easy to roll the cabbage.
2. Grease sides and bottom of Slow Cooker with cooking spray.
3. Add ½ of marinara sauce and set on low settings.
4. In medium bowl, knead with your hands the ground beef, pepper, salt, garlic powder, and onion powder.
5. To assemble, add ¼ cup of meat mixture in one cabbage leaf and roll until meat is secure in the center. Place with seam side down in slow cooker. Repeat the same process for remaining meat and cabbage.
6. Pour remaining marinara sauce on top of cabbage rolls, cover and cook for 5 hours on high.

Nutrition information:

Calories per serving: 900; Carbohydrates: 168.2g; Protein: 51.72g; Fat: 15.87g; Sugar: 67.09g; Sodium: 585mg; Fiber: 47.8g

Corned Beef in Slow Cooker

Points: 5, Serves: 6, Cooking Time: 9 hours, Preparation Time: 8 minutes

Ingredients:

- 2 cups water
- 2-pounds corned beef brisket with seasoning packet
- 1 cabbage, cut into wedges
- 2 onions, chopped

Instructions:

1. In cold running water, rinse corned beef and then dry with paper towels.
2. Place corned beef in slow cooker and sprinkle seasoning packet.
3. Add onions, cabbage, and water.
4. Cover and cook on low for 9 hours.
5. Serve and enjoy.

Nutrition information:

Calories per serving: 314; Carbohydrates: 3.64g; Protein: 22.6g; Fat: 22.57g; Sugar: 1.55g; Sodium: 1843mg; Fiber: 0.6g

Cheesy Pepperoni Breakfast Frittata

Points: 5

Serves: 8

Cooking Time: 8 hours

Preparation Time: 10 minutes

Ingredients:

- Salt and pepper to taste
- 4 tablespoons olive oil
- 12 large eggs
- 1-ounce pepperoni
- ½ cup ricotta cheese
- ½ cup Parmesan cheese

- 5-ounce Mozzarella cheese

Instructions:

1. Grease sides and bottom of Slow Cooker with olive oil.
2. In a large bowl, whisk eggs. Season with pepper and salt.
3. Stir in ricotta cheese and ½ of Mozzarella cheese.
4. Pour egg mixture into slow cooker.
5. Evenly sprinkle remaining mozzarella on top, then followed by Parmesan cheese.
6. Cover and cook for 8 hours on low settings.

Nutrition information:

Calories per serving: 240; Carbs: 3.41g; Protein: 14.11g; Fat: 18.83g; Sugar: 0.74g; Sodium: 333mg; Fiber: 0.4g

Breakfast Burger in Slow Cooker

Points: 4, Serves: 2, Cooking Time: 4 hours, Preparation Time: 15 minutes

Ingredients:

- Pepper and salt to taste
- 1 tablespoon butter
- 2 large eggs
- 2-ounce Pepper jack cheese
- 4-ounce sausage

Instructions:

1. Grease sides and bottom of Slow Cooker with cooking spray.
2. In a medium bowl, break the sausage, season with pepper and salt.
3. Mix well and knead with a fork.
4. Divide into two and form into a Pattie.
5. Divide butter into two pieces and place in slow cooker.
6. Add one Pattie on top of each butter.
7. Cover and cook on high for 3 hours.
8. Turnover Pattie, add cheese on top, and continue cooking for another hour.
9. Serve and enjoy.

Nutrition information:

Calories per serving: 366; Carbohydrates: 8.52g; Protein: 20.65g; Fat: 29.2g; Sugar: 1.39g; Sodium: 729mg; Fiber: 1.9g

Chives and Bacon Omelet

Points: 3, Serves: 1, Cooking Time: 2 hours, Preparation Time: 10 minutes

Ingredients:

- Pepper and salt to taste
- 2 stalks chives
- 1-ounce cheddar cheese
- 2 large eggs
- 2 slices Bacon
- 2 large eggs

Instructions:

1. Grease sides and bottom of Slow Cooker with cooking spray.

2. In a nonstick skillet on medium high fire, cook bacon until crisp. Remove bacon, set aside, and keep warm. Pour bacon fat into slow cooker.
3. In a small bowl, whisk well eggs and season with pepper and salt.
4. Pour egg mixture into slow cooker and cook on high settings for 1.5 hours.
5. Then place bacon and ½ of cheese in middle of egg. Fold egg and turnover to cook for another 30 minutes.
6. To serve, sprinkle chives and remaining cheese and enjoy.

Nutrition information:

Calories per serving: 499; Carbs: 10.17g; Protein: 22.01g; Fat: 41.08g; Sugar: 5.11g; Sodium: 593mg; Fiber: 0.7g

Cheesy Grape Tomato Breakfast Casserole

Points: 4, Serves: 4, Cooking Time: 4 hours, Preparation Time: 10 minutes
Ingredients:
- ½ teaspoon salt
- ½ teaspoon black pepper
- 6 large eggs
- ¾ cup grape tomatoes cut in half
- ¼ cup shredded Parmesan cheese
- ¼ cup Colby cheese
- 1 ½ cups milk

Instructions:
1. Grease sides and bottom of Slow Cooker with cooking spray.
2. In a large bowl, whisk well eggs.
3. Season with salt and pepper.
4. Pour in milk and Colby cheese and whisk well.
5. Pour egg mixture into slow cooker. Evenly space and drop grape tomatoes.
6. Sprinkle Parmesan cheese on top.
7. Cover and cook for 4 hours on high settings, or until set and the sides are lightly browned.

Nutrition information:

Calories per serving: 217; Carbohydrates: 11.74g; Protein: 10.91g; Fat: 14.91g; Sugar: 9.1g; Sodium: 505mg; Fiber: 0.3g

Cauliflower Breakfast Quiche

Points: 2, Serves: 8, Cooking Time: 6 hours, Preparation Time: 20 minutes
Ingredients:
- Pepper and salt to taste
- 12 eggs
- ½ cup milk
- 2 cups cheese
- 1 head cauliflower, shredded
- 2 (5-ounce) packages of pre-cooked breakfast sausages, sliced

Instructions:
1. Grease sides and bottom of Slow Cooker with cooking spray.

2. In a large bowl, lightly beat eggs, pepper and salt.
3. Pour in milk and whisk well.
4. To assemble, place 1/3 of shredded cauliflower in bottom of cooker in an even layer, followed by 1/3 of the sliced sausages, and then 1/3 of the cheese. Season with pepper and salt.
5. Repeat this layering and seasoning process two more times.
6. Then pour in the egg mixture.
7. Cover and cook on low for 6 hours or until set and the sides are lightly browned.

Nutrition information:

Calories per serving: 481; Carbohydrates: 4.66g; Protein: 28.25g; Fat: 38.37g; Sugar: 2.83g; Sodium: 659mg; Fiber: 0.7g

Herbed Egg Casserole for Breakfast

Points: 2,
Serves: 6
Cooking Time: 8 hours
Preparation Time: 10 minutes

Ingredients:
- Pepper and salt to taste
- 8 eggs, whisked
- 1 yellow onion, diced
- 1-pound pork breakfast sausage, broken up
- 2 teaspoons dried basil
- 1 teaspoon dill

Instructions:
1. Grease sides and bottom of Slow Cooker with cooking spray.
2. Add all ingredients in pot, stir to mix.
3. Cover and cook for 8 hours on low settings.

Nutrition information:

Calories per serving: 524; Carbohydrates: 3.16g; Protein: 34.1g; Fat: 40.67g; Sugar: 1.25g; Sodium: 1724mg; Fiber: 0.3g

Bell Pepper-Broccoli Egg Casserole

Points: 3, Serves: 8, Cooking Time: 4 hours, Preparation Time: 15 minutes

Ingredients:
- 1 teaspoon salt
- ½ teaspoon pepper
- 8 eggs
- 6-ounce cheddar cheese
- 1 small head of broccoli, roughly chopped
- 2 bell peppers, chopped roughly
- ¾ cup milk

Instructions:
1. Grease sides and bottom of Slow Cooker with cooking spray.

2. Place ½ of broccoli on bottom of pot, then ½ of bell peppers, and then followed by ½ of cheese. Repeat this process until cheese and broccoli are used up.
3. In a bowl, whisk well eggs, salt, pepper, and milk.
4. Pour egg mixture into pot.
5. Cover and cook on low settings for 4 hours.

Nutrition information:

Calories per serving: 196; Carbohydrates: 7.41g; Protein: 13.82g; Fat: 12.41g; Sugar: 4.5g; Sodium: 647mg; Fiber: 1.3g

Cream Cheese & Mushroom Egg Casserole

Points: 4, Serves: 8, Cooking Time: 2 hours 40 minutes, Preparation Time: 15 minutes

Ingredients:
- Pepper and salt to taste
- 12 medium eggs
- ½ cup milk
- 8-ounce cream cheese, cut into small cubes
- 8-ounce fresh mushrooms, cleaned and sliced
- ½ cup shredded Mexican blend cheese

Instructions:
1. Grease sides and bottom of Slow Cooker with cooking spray.
2. Place a nonstick skillet on medium high fire and cook mushrooms for 10 minutes, until soft.
3. Meanwhile, whisk well eggs. Season with pepper and salt.
4. Pour in milk and whisk well.
5. With a slotted spoon, transfer softened mushrooms into slow cooker and evenly spread on the bottom.
6. Top with cream cheese.
7. Pour in egg mixture.
8. Top with cheese.
9. Cover and cook for 2.5 hours on high settings.

Nutrition information:

Calories per serving: 299; Carbohydrates: 24.22g; Protein: 15.26g; Fat: 17.17g; Sugar: 3.01g; Sodium: 252mg; Fiber: 3.3g

Savory Breakfast Omelet

Points: 2, Serves: 4, Cooking Time: 2 hours, Preparation Time: 15 minutes

Ingredients:
- ¼ teaspoon salt
- Fresh ground pepper, to taste
- ¼ teaspoon garlic powder
- 1 green bell pepper, chopped
- 1 small yellow onion, chopped
- ½ cup chopped tomatoes
- 6 eggs

Instructions:

1. Grease sides and bottom of Slow Cooker with cooking spray.
2. Set on high.
3. Place chopped tomatoes on bottom of pot and spread in an even layer.
4. Spread in an even layer chopped onions, on top of tomatoes, and followed by bell pepper.
5. Cover pot.
6. Meanwhile, in a bowl whisk well eggs. Season with salt, pepper, and garlic powder.
7. Whisk well and then pour into pot.
8. Cover and cook for 2 hours on high.

Nutrition information:

Calories per serving: 236; Carbohydrates: 6.23g; Protein: 14.3g; Fat: 16.89g; Sugar: 3.57g; Sodium: 304mg; Fiber: 0.9g

Egg Casserole with Sausage and Cheese

Points: 3,
Serves 4

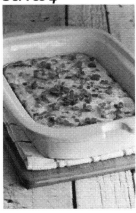

Ingredients
5-6 eggs, beaten until well-combined
Black pepper, fresh ground
1 teaspoons Spike Seasoning
3 ¼ tablespoons sliced green onions
2 ½ teaspoons onions for garnish
12 3/4 tablespoons grated cheddar cheese
1 green pepper, diced
9.6 oz. breakfast sausage links
9 ½ tablespoons cottage cheese, rinsed and drained
1 ¼ teaspoons, divided
Directions
1. Grease a crockpot with non-stick spray or olive oil. Then place cottage cheese into a fine mesh colander. Put the cheese in the sink and rinse with water to wash away the creamy part.
2. In a frying pan, heat a teaspoon of olive oil over medium high heat and cook half of the sausage links until fully browned. Transfer the sausage onto a cutting board to cool down.

3. Now heat a teaspoon of oil and cool the remaining half of the sausage and move it to the cutting board too. You can cook the sausages together if your pan can accommodate them.

4. Heat a teaspoon of oil and brown the pepper pieces for about 2 or 3 minutes. You can cook them directly if you want them somehow crunchy.

5. Once done, cut the sausage links into halves and layer them in the crockpot along with diced or stripped green peppers.

6. Season with cottage cheese and then with the grated cheddar cheese. Top the mixture with sliced onions and top with black pepper and spike seasoning.

7. At this point, beat the eggs until well incorporated and then pour over the cut sausages, cheese and cottage cheese. Distribute the peppers and sausages in the cooking pot using a fork.

8. Close the lid in place and cook the mixture on low heat for 2 hours or more until the cheese is well melted and the eggs are firm in the center.

9. Finally, top with sliced green onions and enjoy the breakfast hot!

Nutritional Information per Serving: Calories 403, Fat 30.0g, Carbs 3.6g, Protein 27.2g

Turkey Crusted Crockpot Breakfast

Points: 4,
Serves 3-4

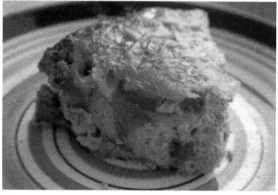

Ingredients
12 tablespoons shredded Monterey Jack cheese
1/4 teaspoons pepper
1/2 cup cottage cheese
3 eggs
1/2 chopped red bell pepper
1/4 chopped onion
1/4 teaspoons Mrs. Dash
1/4 teaspoons fennel seed
1/4 teaspoons sage
1/4 teaspoons onion powder
1/4 teaspoons garlic powder
0.5 pound lean ground turkey

Directions
1. Put the raw turkey meat in the slow cooker and then stir in onion, garlic, fennel, sage and the Mrs. Dash. Stir the ingredients together to blend.
2. Spread the turkey meat over the bottom of the slow cooker using the back of the spoon.
3. Then chop the veggies and now layer them over the poultry meat. In a medium-sized bowl, whisk the eggs.
4. Then stir in cottage cheese, pepper and salt into the whisked eggs and pour the cheese mixture over the veggies and turkey in the slow cooker.
5. Top the ingredients with shredded cheese and cook them on low until set, preferably overnight. If you like it, use low fat turkey sausage as the crust.
Nutritional Information per Serving: Calories 369.9, Fat 22.6g, Carbs 4.4g, Protein 36.2g

Breakfast Stuffed Peppers

Points: 3,

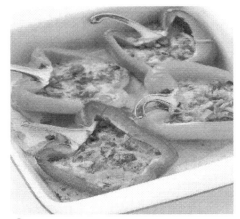

Serves 3

Ingredients
1/4 cup finely chopped ham
6 tablespoons shredded cheddar cheese, divided
2 tablespoons chopped frozen spinach, thawed, squeezed dry
1 tablespoon chopped green onion
Dash teaspoon salt
1/4 cup almond milk
2 eggs
1 1/2 bell peppers, halved and seeded
Directions
1. Line a crockpot with tin foil then add the peppers and fill with the rest of the ingredients.
2. Cook on low heat for about 3 to 4 hours or until eggs are cooked through.
Nutritional Information per Serving: Calories 164, Fat 10g, Carbs 6g, Protein 11g

Overnight Breakfast Casserole

Points: 5,
Serves 4-5

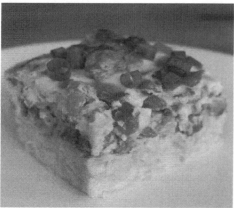

Ingredients
Dash teaspoon cracked black pepper
Dash teaspoon dry mustard
1/2 teaspoon sea salt
2 tablespoons full-fat coconut milk
3 ¼ tablespoons almond milk
6-7 large eggs, beaten
1 orange bell pepper, seeded and diced
1 red bell pepper, seeded and diced
0.4 pound rutabagas, peeled and shredded
3 ¼ tablespoons yellow onion, diced
2.4 ounces bacon, chopped
3.2 ounce bulk breakfast sausage, crumbled
Softened ghee, to greasing the crockpot
Green onions, for garnish

Directions
1. First grease the bottom and sides of a crockpot using softened ghee or palm shortening.
2. Then cook the onion, bacon and the sausage in the slow cooker until the onion is softened and the sausage browned, or for about 10 to 12 minutes.
3. Discard any excess fat. Now add in shredded rutabaga in the crockpot and press them down gently.
4. Add in the onion and meat mixture and bell peppers on top.
5. In a separate bowl, whisk together eggs, mustard, salt, milk and pepper. Pour into the crockpot.
6. Cook the mixture on low for 6 to 8 hours or until cooked through.

Nutritional Information per Serving: Calories 375, Fat 16.3g, Carb 7.5g, Protein 18.8g

Crock Pot Mexican Breakfast Casserole

Points: 5,
Servings 4

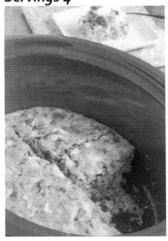

Ingredients
¼ cup Pepper Jack cheese
¼ cup coconut milk
4 eggs
¼ cup salsa
Dash teaspoon pepper
Dash teaspoon salt
1/2 teaspoon chili powder
1/2 teaspoon cumin
1/8 teaspoon coriander
1/8 teaspoon garlic powder
4.75 ounces Jones Dairy Farm Pork Sausage Roll
Avocado salsa, sour cream and cilantro: optional
Directions
1. First cook the pork sausage in a large skillet over medium heat until it's no longer pink.
2. Season and add salsa then set aside to slightly cool down.
3. In a separate bowl, whisk the coconut milk with eggs then add in pork to the eggs.
4. Now add in Jack cheese and stir to blend. Grease the bottom of a slow cooker and pour in the egg mixture.
5. Finally cook on low for 5 hours or high for 2 ½ hours. Serve topped with preferred toppings.
Nutritional Information per Serving: Calories 320, Fat 24.1g, Carbs 5.2g, Protein 17.9g

Cauliflower Breakfast Casserole

Points: 4,
Serves 3

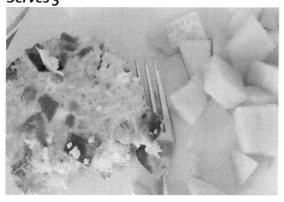

Ingredients
1 cup of shredded cheddar cheese
4 slices of low sodium, all natural turkey bacon, cooked and diced
1/2 small bell pepper, diced
1/2 small onion, diced
Salt and pepper
1/2 head cauliflower
1/4 teaspoon pepper
1/2 teaspoon Himalayan salt
1/8 teaspoon dry mustard
2 tablespoons unsweetened almond milk
4 large eggs

Directions
1. Coat a slow cooker with coconut oil or olive oil spray and set aside.
2. Then mix together dry mustard, eggs, salt, almond milk and pepper in a large bowl.
3. Put around 1/3 of the cauliflower in the bottom of the crockpot and top with one third of the bell pepper and onion.
4. Season with pepper and salt, and top with one third of the cheese and one third of the bacon. Repeat the layers two more rounds.
5. At this point, pour the egg mixture over the layers of the ingredients in the crockpot.
6. Cook until the eggs are set and browned at the top, for about 5-7 hours or so. Serve and enjoy.

Nutritional Information per Serving: Calories 324.5, Fat 22.5g, Carbs 7.5g, Protein 22.6g

Crock Pot Cauliflower Breakfast

Points: 2,
Serves 4

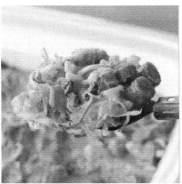

Ingredients
4 oz. Cheddar cheese
1/8 teaspoon salt
3 eggs
1/2 leek, cut into quarter inch half-moon slices
6 cooked sausage links, cut into quarter inch rounds
2.5 oz. cremini mushrooms, finely diced
1/8 teaspoon salt
5 oz. cauliflower florets

Directions
1. Grease a crockpot with cooking spray and set aside. Meanwhile add pieces of the cauliflower to a heat-safe bowl along with salt.
2. Add water to the bowl and fill it to entirely cover the cauliflower, and put it in the microwave to cook for about 8 minutes.
3. As it cooks, be preparing the leeks, sausage and mushrooms. Then drain off the liquid from the half cooked cauliflower and add it to the crockpot.
4. Evenly distribute the sausage and mushrooms pieces on the cauliflower and set aside.
5. Now whisk together salt and eggs in a bowl and carefully stir in cleaned leeks. Slowly stir in half of the cheese and reserve the other half.
6. Then pour the egg mixture uniformly over the cauliflower pieces, sausage and the mushrooms.
7. Cover the ingredients and cook on high for about 2 to 3 hours, or until the eggs puff up.
8. At this point, sprinkle the rest of the cheese over the top and allow it to melt. Then slice the casserole and enjoy. Season the dish with salt and pepper if you like.

Nutritional Information per Serving: Calories 356.5, Fat 29.9g, Carbs 4.5g, Protein 18.9g

Slow Cooker Breakfast Meatloaf

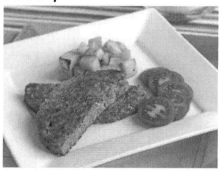

Ingredients

1/2 teaspoon sea salt

1/2 teaspoon paprika

1/2 teaspoon black pepper

1 teaspoon dried thyme

1 teaspoon ground sage

1 teaspoon red pepper flakes

1 teaspoon dried oregano

1 teaspoon fennel seeds, ground

1/2 garlic powder

4 tablespoons almond flour

1 egg

1 lb. ground pork

1 cup diced onion

1/2 tablespoon coconut oil

Directions

1. At medium-low heat, soften the onion in a tablespoon of oil until transparent. Then remove from heat and let cool.

2. Add all the ingredients to a large bowl apart from the ground pork. Stir or whisk to blend.

3. Add in the softened onions and the ground pork to the bowl and combine the ingredients manually using your hands.

4. Then pick the meat mixture and put it in the center of the crockpot's insert. Shape it into a loaf and position it half an inch from the sides of the insert.

5. Once done, pat the top the loaf and close the crockpot's lid. Cook the meatloaf on low for 3 hours, or until the internal temperature is 150 degrees F.

6. Then let the meatloaf cool for up to 30 minutes after turning off the crockpot and removing the lid to make it easier to remove the meatloaf. Move to a separate dish.

7. You can serve immediately or keep it refrigerated overnight and serve for breakfast. To serve, simply reheat the slices at medium low heat for a minute or two.

Nutritional Information per Serving: Calories 412.6, Fat 28.7g, Carbs 5.0g, Protein 32.5g

Frittata with Artichoke Hearts

Points: 4,
Serves 3

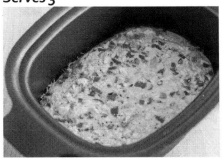

Ingredients
Black pepper, fresh-ground
1/2 teaspoon all-purpose seasoning
2 oz. crumbled Feta cheese
4 eggs, beaten well
2 tablespoons cup sliced green onions
1/2 jar (12 oz.) roasted red peppers, chopped
1/2 (14 oz.) can artichoke hearts pieces, drained
1 tablespoon chopped parsley, optional

Directions
1. Place the artichoke hearts into a colander that is placed in the sink and let drain well.
2. Once drained, crumble the feta and slice the green onions. Meanwhile, lightly coat a Crockpot with non-stick spray.
3. Move the artichokes to a cutting board and pour the peppers into the colander.
4. Cut the artichokes into pieces and place them into the slow cooker insert.
5. Then cut the peppers into ½-inch squares and place them in the Crockpot. Add in green onions.
6. At this point, beat the yolks and egg whites until well combined. Pour the egg mixture over the veggies in the Crockpot.
7. Stir gently using a fork to well distribute sliced green onions, red pepper pieces and artichoke pieces.
8. Sprinkle the feta over the top and season with the ground pepper and all-purpose seasoning.
9. Cook for about 2-3 hours or until the cheese has melted and the eggs are firm.
10. Finally cut the frittata in pieces while still in the Crockpot. Serve it hot, sprinkled with parsley if you like.

Nutritional Information per Serving: Calories 185, Fat 10g, Protein 13g, Carbs 9g

Freestyle Breakfast Frittata

Points: 4,
Serves 3

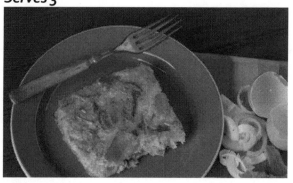

Ingredients
2/3 cups cook sausage, breakfast
1/2 teaspoon sea salt
1/4 teaspoons black pepper
4 individual beat eggs
2 tablespoons dice onion, red
¾ cups dice bell pepper, red
3 ounce drain spinach, frozen
Directions
1. Mix together spinach, sea salt, black pepper, eggs, red onions, sausage and red pepper in an oil-greased Crockpot.
2. Cover and cook for 2-3 hours on low or until set.
3. In case you'd like to freeze the frittata, cool it for a moment then cut into equal-sized portions.
4. Then divide it among 1 gallon freezer bags and keep it frozen until ready to serve.
Nutritional Information per Serving: 238 Calories, 3g Carbs, 16g Fat, 20g Protein

Cheese and Mushroom Strata

Points: 5,
Serves 3
Ingredients
1/8 teaspoon salt
1/2 tablespoon Dijon
1 tablespoon thyme, finely chopped
1 1/4 cups milk
4 eggs
1 cup grated gruyere cheese
friendly bread, cut into 1-inch pieces
2 1/2 thick slices
½ -227g package cremini mushrooms, sliced

Olive oil

1/2 tablespoon

Directions

1. Over medium-high heat, melt oil in a non-stick frying pan. Add in mushrooms and cook for about 5-6 minutes, or until the mushrooms are tender and their liquid evaporated.

2. Using a large piece of coil, line the bottoms and sides of a Crockpot. Lightly coat with oil

3. Cover the bottom with a third of the bread then scatter the mushrooms over the bread.

4. Sprinkle the mixture with a third of the cheese, and then add half of the remaining bread, and the rest of mushrooms and cheese. Add the remaining bread on top.

5. At this point, beat eggs with Dijon, thyme and milk in a large bowl. Pour the mixture over the bread and season with fresh pepper.

6. Carefully press down the bread to soak into the mixture and top with cheese. Cook on low for 8 hours.

7. Once set, open the lid and allow to stand for 15 minutes. Remove the foil that holds the strata using oven mitts.

8. Move the dish to a serving dish and serve with a favorite salad.

Nutritional Information per Serving: Calories 191, Carbs 20g, Protein 14g, Fat 5g

Spinach and Mozzarella Frittata

Points: 4,
Serves 3

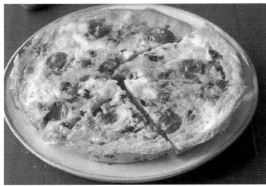

Ingredients

1/2 Roma tomato, diced

Salt to taste

1/2 cup chopped baby spinach, without stems

1/8 teaspoon white pepper

1/8 teaspoon black pepper

1 tablespoon coconut milk

2 egg whites

2 eggs

1/2 cup 2% shredded mozzarella cheese, divided

1/4 cup diced onion

1/2 tablespoon extra-virgin olive oil

Directions

1. Add oil to a small skillet and sauté the onion for around 5 minutes. Once tender, remove from the skillet and set aside.

2. With non-stick cooking spray, coat a slow cooker and set aside.

3. Mix together ¾ of the cheese, sautéed onion and the rest of the ingredients. Whisk to combine and transfer to the Crockpot.

4. Now sprinkle with the remaining mozzarella on top of the mixture. Cook the contents on low for 1 hour to 1 ½ hours while covered.

5. As soon as the eggs are set, remove from the cooker and serve.

Nutritional Information per Serving: Carbs: 4g, Calories: 139, Fat: 8g, Protein: 12g

Sausage & Egg Breakfast Casserole

Points: 5,

Serves 3

Ingredients

1/8 teaspoon pepper

1/4 teaspoon salt

1 clove garlic, minced

6 tablespoons (3 ounce) whipping cream

5 eggs

1/2 cup shredded Cheddar, divided

6-oz sausage, cooked and sliced

1/2 medium head broccoli, chopped

Directions

1. With oil, grease your Crockpot then layer half of the broccoli, half of the cheese and half of the sausage into it.

2. Repeat the layering with the rest of broccoli, sausage and cheese.

3. Then whisk eggs, garlic, whipping cream, salt and pepper until well blended. Pour over the sausage and cheese layers.

4. Cover the Crockpot and cook the ingredients for 2-3 hours on high or 4-5 hours on low.

5. As soon as the contents are set in the center and browned on the edges, serve.

Nutritional Information per Serving: Carbs: 5.39g, Calories: 484, fat: 38.86g Protein: 26.13g

Cheese Shrimp and Cauliflower Grits

Points: 5,
Serves 4

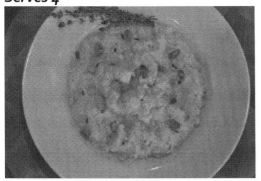

Ingredients

2 pounds raw shrimp

½ cup grated parmesan cheese

4 ounces light cream cheese

1 cup light sharp cheddar cheese

Salt and pepper to taste

2 teaspoons fresh thyme, chopped

1 tablespoon onion powder

1 tablespoon garlic powder

1 ½ cups cauliflower "grits"

6 cups chicken broth or stock

Cheese for garnish

Scallions or chives, optional

1/2 teaspoon hot sauce, optional

Directions

1. Mix together grits and chicken broth in a Crockpot. Add in the rest of the ingredients apart from green onions and shrimp.

2. Cook for 3 hours on low then add in ½ cup of cream or half and half along with the shrimp.

3. Cook for another 30 minutes or up to one hour to fully cook the fish.

4. Once done, garnish with cheese, chives and green onions if desired.

Nutritional Information per Serving: Calories 538.0, Fat 27.7g, Carbs 8.8g, Protein 62.8g

Crockpot Breakfast Casserole

Points: 5,
Serves: 4

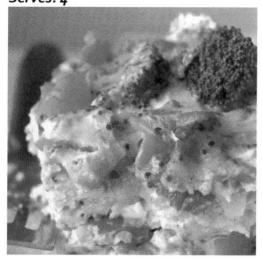

Ingredients
3 oz. cheddar cheese
½ small head of broccoli, chopped
1 bell pepper, chopped
1/4 onion, chopped
2 strips cooked bacon, optional
15 oz. rutabagas
1/4 teaspoon pepper
1/2 teaspoon salt
1/4 teaspoon garlic salt
2 teaspoon stone mustard, ground
3 ounce cup of coconut milk
2 egg whites
4 eggs
Directions
1. Whisk together whole eggs, milk, egg whites, garlic, mustard, salt and pepper in a medium bowl and set aside.
2. Grease your slow cooker with oil then put half of the hash browns on the bottom.
3. Then layer half amounts of each of the following: bacon, bell peppers, chopped onion, broccoli and cheese.
4. Add in the rest of the hash browns, top with the remaining veggies, bacon and the cheese. Then pour the egg mixture on top.
5. Then cover the cooker and let cook for 4 hours on low heat. Serve it while hot.
Nutritional Information per Serving: Calories 187.4, Fat 11.9g, Carbs 6.7g, Protein 13.g

Sausage and Pepper Breakfast Hash

Points: 5,
Serves 4

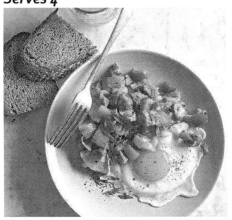

Ingredients

1 teaspoons snipped fresh parsley

3 ¼ tablespoons shredded Swiss cheese

3/4 cups sweet peppers, chopped

2 tablespoon reduced-sodium chicken broth

1/4 teaspoon ground black pepper

1 teaspoon dried thyme, crushed

3/4 pounds of chopped daikon

Nonstick cooking spray

3/4 cups sliced sweet onion

1/2 teaspoon olive oil

1/2 12-ounce package smoked chicken sausage with apple, cooked

Directions

1. Cook the sausage in a non-stick skillet for 5 minutes over medium heat. Once browned, remove from the skillet.

2. Heat oil in the skillet over medium-low heat. Then cook the onion until tender or until it begins to brown, for about 5 minutes, while stirring.

3. Meanwhile, coat the bottom of a Crockpot with cooking spray and add in sausage, daikon or rutabagas, onion, black pepper and thyme.

4. Pour broth over the ingredients then cover the slow cooker. Cook for 2 ½ to 3 hours on high heat or 5-6 hours on low.

5. Then stir in the sweet peppers and sprinkle with cheese if you like. In case you cooked under low heat, turn the Crockpot to high heat.

6. Cover and cook for another 15 minutes then serve with a slotted spoon. Sprinkle with parsley or tarragon.

Nutritional Information Per Serving: Calories 131, 18 g carbs, 3 g fat, 7 g proteins

Feta-Kale Egg Casserole

Points: 3, Serves: 6, Cooking Time: 3 hours 4 minutes, Preparation Time: 15 minutes

Ingredients:
- Salt and pepper to taste
- 5-ounce baby kale
- ¼ cup sliced green onion
- 5-ounce crumbled Feta cheese
- 8 eggs
- 1 cup low-fat sour cream

Instructions:
1. Grease sides and bottom of Slow Cooker with cooking spray.
2. Place a nonstick skillet on medium high fire and grease with cooking spray.
3. Sauté kale until it is flat and softened, around 4 minutes.
4. In a large bowl, beat eggs and season with pepper and salt.
5. Mix in kale, green onion and feta cheese.
6. Pour into pot, cover, and cook on low for 3 hours.
7. To serve, place a dollop of sour cream on top of a slice of the dish.

Nutrition information:

Calories per serving: 331; Carbohydrates: 8.52g; Protein: 19.64g; Fat: 24.24g; Sugar: 5.2g; Sodium: mg; Fiber: 1g

Mexican Breakfast Frittata

Points: 4

Serves: 6

Cooking Time: 3 hours minutes

Preparation Time: 8 minutes

Ingredients:
- ½ teaspoon pepper
- 9 large eggs
- 8-ounce shredded low-fat Cheddar cheese
- 1 teaspoon Mexican oregano
- 1 small onion, diced
- 1 cup salsa

Instructions:
1. Grease sides and bottom of Slow Cooker with cooking spray.
2. Set on high settings.
3. In large bowl, whisk well and season with pepper.
4. Mix in oregano, cheese, and onion.
5. Pour into pot.
6. Cover and cook on low for 3 hours.
7. To serve, add a dollop of salsa on each slice of frittata.

Nutrition information:

Calories per serving: 167; Carbohydrates: 6.11g; Protein: 14.13g; Fat: 9.51g; Sugar: 2.74g; Sodium: 649mg; Fiber: 1.1g

Cheesy Shrimp Breakfast Casserole

Points: 3, Serves: 4, Cooking Time: 3 hours, Preparation Time: 15 minutes

Ingredients:
- Salt and pepper to taste
- 1-pound raw shrimp, peeled and deveined
- 6 large eggs
- 1 cup sharp cheddar cheese, shredded
- 4-ounces cream cheese, chopped
- ½ cup milk

Instructions:
1. Grease sides and bottom of Slow Cooker with cooking spray.
2. In a large bowl, whisk well eggs.
3. Season with pepper and salt.
4. Stir in milk and ½ of cheddar cheese.
5. Stir in cream cheese and shrimp.
6. Pour into pot.
7. Cover and cook in slow cooker for 2 hours on high settings.
8. Uncover and sprinkle cheese on top and cook for another 30 to 60 minutes or until the middle of the casserole is set.

Nutrition information:

Calories per serving: 331; Carbohydrates: 8.52g; Protein: 19.64g; Fat: 24.24g; Sugar: 5.2g; Sodium: 507mg; Fiber: 1g

Egg and Shrimp Breakfast Casserole

Points: 3, Serves: 4, Cooking Time: 3 hours, Preparation Time: 5 minutes

Ingredients:
- Pepper and salt to taste
- 6 eggs
- 1-pound raw shrimp, peeled and deveined
- 2 stalks green onions, chopped

Instructions:
1. Grease sides and bottom of Slow Cooker with cooking spray.
2. Set on High settings.
3. Place ½ of shrimp on bottom of pot and evenly spread.
4. Meanwhile, in bowl whisk eggs. Season with pepper and salt.
5. Pour egg mixture in pot.
6. Gently sprinkle remaining half of shrimp on top of eggs.
7. Cover and cook for 2 hours.
8. Then sprinkle green onions on top.
9. Continue cooking until center is set, around 30 to 60 minutes more.

Nutrition information:

Calories per serving: 312; Carbohydrates: 2.59g; Protein: 36.83g; Fat: 16.02g; Sugar: 1.55g; Sodium: 1114mg; Fiber: 0.2g

Points: 5,
Serves 4

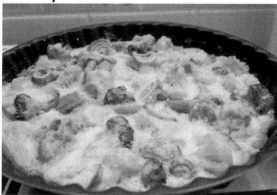

Ingredients
1/3 cup almond milk
4 eggs
1/2 cup shredded Cheddar cheese
1/3 cup green bell pepper, diced
1/3 pound diced ham
1/3 cup chopped onion
2/3 pound cauliflower

Directions
1. Add or layer the ingredients in a slow cooker starting with tater torts, then ham, onions, green pepper and finally the cheese. Make another two layers from taters to cheese.
2. Beat eggs and milk in a separate bowl. Season the egg mixture with salt and pepper. Then pour the mixture over the ingredients in the slow cooker.
3. Cover and cook for 10-12 hours on low heat.

Nutritional Information per Serving: Calories 206.3, Fat 11.4g, Carbs 8.1g, Protein 18.3g

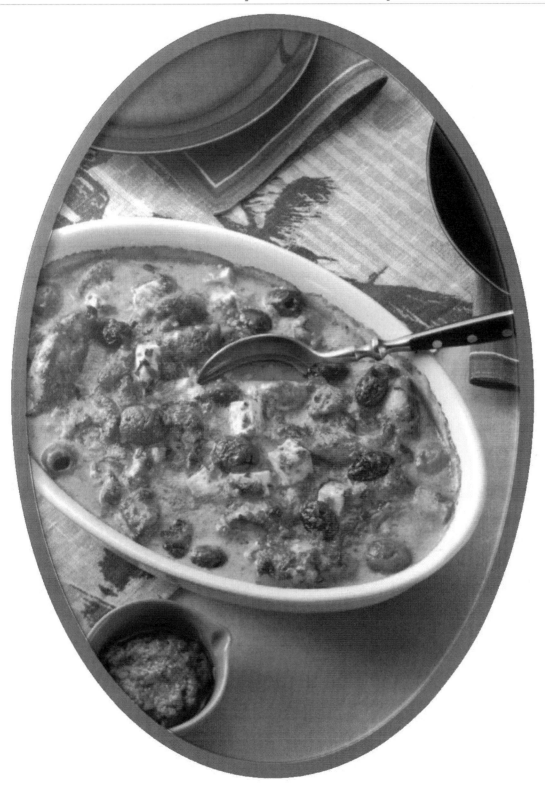

Freestyle Shrimp Fra Diavolo

Points: 4,
Serves 4
 Ingredients
1/4 pound medium-size shrimp, shelled
1/2 teaspoon black pepper, freshly ground
1 tablespoon Italian parsley, minced
1 (14.5-ounce) can fire-roasted tomatoes, diced
1 teaspoon red pepper flakes
3-5 cloves of garlic, minced
1 medium onion, diced
1 teaspoon avocado oil
Directions
1. In a non-stick frying pan, heat some oil over medium heat.
2. Then sauté garlic, onion and pepper flakes until the onion has softened and is translucent. This should take about 8 to 10 minutes.
3. Now add black pepper, parsley, tomatoes and onion mixture to a slow cooker. Stir to blend then cook for 2 to 3 hours, on low heat.
4. Add in shrimp, stir and cover. Cook until cooked through, or for 15 minutes on high heat.
5. Serve.
Nutritional Information per Serving: Calories 173.7, Fat 3.3g, Carbs 9.9g, Protein 24.3g

Hawaiian Style Slow Cooked Pork

Serves: 8, Cooking Time: 12 hours, Preparation Time: 15 minutes
Ingredients:
- 5 peeled garlic cloves
- 1 ½ tablespoons Alaea Red Hawaiian Coarse Sea Salt
- 5-pound Boston Butt roast, with bone
- 3 slices bacon

Instructions:
1. In slow cooker, place bacon on bottom of pot.
2. Rub salt all over the pork.
3. Cut 5 short but deep slits in the meat and stick in 1 garlic clove in each slit.
4. Place pork on top of bacon slices.
5. Cover and cook on low for 10 to 12 hours.
6. Once pork butt is tender, remove from pot and transfer to a bowl.
7. Shred with two forks, serve and enjoy.
8. Discard sauce because this will be too salty.

Nutrition information:

Calories per serving: 800; Carbohydrates: 0.81g; Protein: 72.44g; Fat: 53.99g; Sugar: 0.17g; Sodium: 218mg; Fiber: 0.1g

Salsa-Pineapple Chicken

Points: 6, Serves: 8, Cooking Time: 6 hours, Preparation Time: 15 minutes

Ingredients:

- 2 20-ounce can pineapple chunks in 100% juice
- 1 16-ounce jar tomato salsa
- 2-pounds boneless, skinless chicken breasts

Instructions:

1. Grease sides and bottom of Slow Cooker with cooking spray.
2. Place chicken breasts on bottom of pot.
3. Pour in pineapples and its juice into pot.
4. Add salsa and stir to mix well and cover chicken.
5. Cover and cook on low settings for 6 hours.

Nutrition information:

Calories per serving: 291; Carbohydrates: 47.63g; Protein: 11.66g; Fat: 6.71g; Sugar: 26.56g; Sodium: 317mg; Fiber: 3.2g

Garlicky and Lemony Chicken

Points: 5, Serves: 4, Cooking Time: 4 hours, Preparation Time: 10 minutes

Ingredients:

- Salt and pepper to taste
- 2 sprigs of fresh rosemary
- 1 whole chicken, around 4-pounds
- 2 heads of garlic
- 2 lemons

Instructions:

1. Grease sides and bottom of Slow Cooker with cooking spray.
2. Slice each head of garlic across in half and place 3 slices on bottom of pot.
3. Slice one lemon into 4 equal round slices and place on bottom of pot, right beside the garlic.
4. Set on high.
5. Slice lemon into half. Squeeze ½ of the lemon all over the chicken.
6. Season chicken generously with salt and pepper inside and out.
7. Inside the chicken place one half of the remaining garlic and 1 sprig of rosemary.
8. Place chicken on top of lemon and garlic on slow cooker.
9. Top chicken with rosemary and remaining garlic.
10. Then slice the remaining lemon into thin and round slices and place on top of chicken.
11. Cover and cook for 4 hours or until chicken has reached and internal temperature of 165-degrees Fahrenheit.

Nutrition information:

Calories per serving: 295; Carbohydrates: 6.03g; Protein: 49.34g; Fat: 7.32g; Sugar: 1.19g; Sodium: 184mg; Fiber: 2.2g

White Chili Chicken in Slow Cooker

Points: 6, Serves: 4, Cooking Time: 8 hours, Preparation Time: 5 minutes

Ingredients:

- 2 cups salsa Verde
- 2 15-ounce cans Great Northern beans, drained
- 6 chicken thighs, boneless and skinless, cut into quarters
- 6 cups chicken broth

Instructions:

1. Grease sides and bottom of Slow Cooker with cooking spray.
2. Place chicken in bottom of pot.
3. Add cumin, salsa Verde, beans, and broth.
4. Cover and cook for 8 hours.
5. Remove chicken and shred with two forks. Return to pot.
6. Mix well.
7. Serve and enjoy

Nutrition information:

Calories per serving: 1429; Carbohydrates: 142.61g; Protein: 98.05g; Fat: 52.36g; Sugar: 10.61g; Sodium: 2370mg; Fiber: 45.2g

Java Flavor Roast Beef

Points: 7, Serves: 4, Cooking Time: 8 hours 5 minutes, Preparation Time: 10 minutes

Ingredients:

- ¼ water
- ¾ teaspoon salt
- 1 ½ teaspoons salt
- 5 garlic cloves, minced
- 1 boneless beef chuck roast, around 3-pounds
- 2 tablespoons cornstarch
- 1 ½ cup strong brewed coffee

Instructions:

1. Grease sides and bottom of Slow Cooker with cooking spray.
2. Season meat with pepper, salt, and garlic.
3. Place meat in slow cooker and pour brewed coffee.
4. Cover and cook for 10 hours on low.
5. Once done, transfer meat to a serving plate and keep warm.
6. In a medium pot, place on medium-high fire, pour all sauces from slow cooker.
7. In a small bowl, whisk well cornstarch and water.
8. Once sauce in pot is boiling, lower fire and slowly pour in cornstarch mixture while continuously stirring sauce.
9. Continue whisking and cooking until sauce is thickened around 3 minutes.

Nutrition information:

Calories per serving: 300; Carbohydrates: 4.89g; Protein: 40.93g; Fat: 12.92g; Sugar: 0.04g; Sodium: 1433mg; Fiber: 0.1g

Pork Roast with Apple and Garlic

Points: 7, Serves: 6
Cooking Time: 8 hours
Preparation Time: 10 minutes

Ingredients:

- ½ cup water
- 1 teaspoons pepper
- 1 teaspoon salt
- 2 ½ teaspoons minced garlic
- 1 tablespoons dried parsley flakes
- 1 medium apple, cored and sliced thinly
- 1 boneless pork loin roast, around 3-pounds

Instructions:

1. Cut the pork in half.
2. Grease sides and bottom of Slow Cooker with cooking spray.
3. Add all ingredient sin pot except for roast and mix well.
4. Place roast in pot.
5. Cover and cook for 10 hours on low.

Nutrition information:

Calories per serving: 504; Carbohydrates: 5.31g; Protein: 82.23g; Fat: 14.93g; Sugar: 3.55g; Sodium: 569mg; Fiber: 0.9g

Easy Ham in Slow Cooker

Points: 6,
Serves: 15
Cooking Time: 8 hours
Preparation Time: 15 minutes

Ingredients:

- 1 fully cooked boneless ham, cut in half, around 6 pounds
- 1 teaspoon ground mustard
- 1 teaspoon prepared horseradish
- 1 20-ounce can of pineapple
- 1 cup water

Instructions:

1. Add all ingredients in slow cooker.
2. Cover and cook for 8 hours.
3. Slice and serve.

Nutrition information:

Calories per serving: 448; Carbohydrates: 16.82g; Protein: 49.57g; Fat: 18.81g; Sugar: 16.52g; Sodium: 143mg; Fiber: 0.3g

Low Carbs Old-Style Beef Stew

Points: 7

Serves: 5

Cooking Time: 6 hours minutes

Preparation Time: 20 minutes

Ingredients:

● 1 cup water

● 1 ½-pounds beef stew meat, cubed into 1-inch squares

● 16-ounce fresh cremini mushrooms

● 3 medium tomatoes, chopped

● 1 envelope reduced sodium onion soup mix

Instructions:

1. Add all ingredients in slow cooker.
2. Cover and cook on low settings for 6 hours.
3. Serve and enjoy.

Nutrition information:

Calories per serving: 551; Carbohydrates: 71.52g; Protein: 58.15g; Fat: 7.82g; Sugar: 4.01g; Sodium: 522mg; Fiber: 11.4g

Slow Cooker Mexican Ground Beef

Points: 6

Serves: 6

Cooking Time: 3 hours

Preparation Time: 15 minutes

Ingredients:

● 1 ½-pounds ground beef

● 2 cups shredded cheddar cheese

● 1 envelope taco seasoning

● 1 can 10.75-ounce condensed tomato soup

● 1 cup sour cream

Instructions:

1. Grease sides and bottom of Slow Cooker with cooking spray.
2. Set on high.
3. On nonstick skillet placed on medium high fire, cook ground beef for 5-minutes. Transfer to slow cooker.
4. Add can of tomato soup and taco seasoning and mix well.
5. Sprinkle cheese on top.
6. Cover and cook for 2 hours.
7. To serve, add a dollop of sour cream on each e=serving and enjoy.

Nutrition information:

Calories per serving: 496; Carbohydrates: 3.88g; Protein: 39.07g; Fat: 35.19g; Sugar: 0.41g; Sodium: 402mg; Fiber: 0.1g

Pork Chops with French Onion Sauce

Points: 7, Serves: 4, Cooking Time: 4 hours, Preparation Time: 5 minutes

Ingredients:

- ½ cup sour cream
- 1 can Campbell's French Onion Soup, 10.5-ounce
- 1 can Campbell's chicken broth, 10.5-ounce
- 4 boneless center cut pork loin chops

Instructions:

1. Mix well the first three ingredient inside the slow cooker.
2. Add the chops.
3. Cover and cook on high settings for 4 hours.

Nutrition information:

Calories per serving: 311; Carbohydrates: 11.04g; Protein: 43.88g; Fat: 10.05g; Sugar: 2.56g; Sodium: 737mg; Fiber: 1g

Crock Pot Luau Pork with Cauliflower Rice

Points: 6
Servings: 4

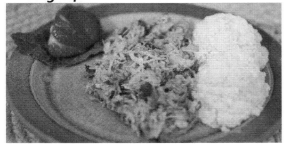

Ingredients

1 tablespoon hickory liquid smoke, plain
3 cloves garlic minced.
3/4 tablespoon sea salt
2 slices Bacon hickory smoked, nitrate free.
1 1/2 lb. pork roast, shoulder or butt
Cauli Rice:
1/8 teaspoon sea salt
8 teaspoons garlic powder
1 tablespoon homemade chicken broth
1 1/2 cups cauliflower

Directions

1. Set the slow cooker to high heat setting, then line the bottom with bacon slices. Sprinkle with garlic to cover the raw meat.
2. Poke and stab all over the meat using a sharp knife. Pour a sufficient amount of sea salt into a bowl and then rub it over the meat.
3. Put the roast in the slow cooker, fat side down. Add some liquid smoke if you like it over the meat and cover the cooker.

4. Cook the roast for 4 to 6 hours in high heat settings, then for a further 2 hours on low heat.

5. Once cooked through, pull apart the roast in the slow cooker using a fork to check if it falls apart easily.

6. Then stir in bacon and shredded bacon in the cooking pot and cover. Cook for about 30 minutes on low heat.

7. To make the cauliflower rice, steam it for 20 minute or microwave for 5 minutes.

8. Then put cooled cauli rice in a blender along with sea salt, garlic and homemade chicken broth. Blend to achieve rice consistency.

9. Once done, put a scoop of the cauliflower rice on a plate and op with a scoop of shredded pork.

10. Serve warm.

Nutritional Information per Serving: Calories 182, Fat 13g, Carbs 2g, Protein 14g

Spinach Artichoke Chicken

Points: 7

Serves 4

Ingredients

1 cup cherry tomatoes, chopped

6- 8 artichoke hearts from a jar, drained and chopped

4 tablespoons parmesan cheese, shredded

4 tablespoons cream cheese, reduced-fat

1/4 sweet onion, finely chopped

3 cloves fresh garlic, chopped

4 (6-8 ounce) whole chicken breasts

1 cup chicken broth

8 cups loosely packed spinach, chopped

Salt

Pepper

Directions

1. In a Crockpot, add chicken breast, chicken broth and spinach then sprinkle with salt, pepper and garlic.

2. Cook on high for 4-6 hours or low for 6-8 hours.

3. Transfer the chicken breast on serving platters. Stir in artichokes, parmesan cheese and cream cheese into the cooker until creamy.

4. Spoon the cheese sauce over the chicken.

5. To serve, top with the tomatoes and sprinkle some parmesan cheese if you like.

Nutritional Information per Serving: Carbs: 14g, Calories: 246, Fat: 6g, Protein: 35g

Points: 8
Serves 4

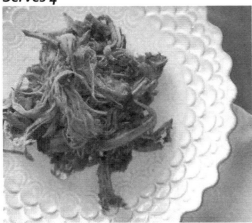

Ingredients
2 tablespoons coconut vinegar
1 1/2 cups bone broth
1/4 large sweet onion, chopped
1 1/2 tablespoons tomato paste
1/8 teaspoon sea salt
1/4 teaspoon ground cinnamon
1/2 teaspoon cardamom powder
1/2 teaspoon cumin powder
1/4 teaspoon whole peppercorns
1/2 teaspoon whole cloves
1/2 teaspoon whole fennel seeds
Sea salt and pepper
1 1/2 lbs. grass fed beef brisket

Directions
1. Season both sides of the brisket with pepper and salt.
2. Then mix together peppercorns, cloves and fennel seeds in a pestle and mortar and grind to obtain fine powder.
3. Move the mixture to a blender or food processor along with onion and tomato paste.
4. Puree until smooth then add in vinegar and broth. Puree again to obtain a smooth sauce.
5. At this point, put the brisket in the crockpot and pour the sauce over it. Set the crockpot to low and cook the brisket for 7 to 8 hours.
6. Once cooked through, shred with a fork and serve.

Nutritional Information per Serving: Calories 423.7, Fat 22.0g, Carb 2.3g, Protein 51.3g

Crockpot Buffalo Chicken

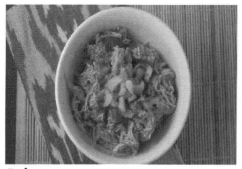

Points: 5

Serves: 3

Ingredients

3/4 cups of chicken broth

1 clove of garlic

1/2 small onion (quartered)

1 whole stalk of celery

1 whole carrot or radish

1 pound of boneless chicken

Salt and pepper to taste

5 1/3 tablespoon of buffalo sauce

1 tablespoons of butter

Directions

1. To a slow cooker, add the chicken breasts, whole garlic cloves, onions, whole carrots, the celery ribs, whole garlic and chicken broth.

2. Use the salt and pepper to season.

3. Then set your Crockpot on high heat and cook for 4 hours.

4. Discard everything except the 1/3 cup of cooking liquid and the veggies.

5. Now use two forks to shred the chicken into small pieces. If you wish to use the buffalo sauce and butter, add it in then let it cook for 15 extra minutes.

Nutritional Information per Serving: Calories 154.4g, Protein 33.9g, Carbs 8.1g, Fat 3.5g

Tasty Mississippi Roast

Points: 7

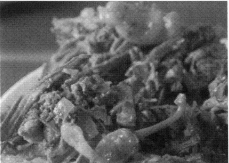

Serves: 4

Ingredients

2 tablespoon butter

1/2 cup pepperoncini

Black pepper, freshly ground

Kosher salt

2 lb. boneless beef chuck roast

1/2 packet ranch seasoning

1/4 large onion, finely chopped

1/4 cup beef broth

Directions

1. Mix together onion, ranch seasoning and beef broth in the Crockpot until blended.

2. Add in chuck roast and season with pepper and salt. Add butter and pepperoncini.

3. Cover and cook at low heat for 6 to 8 hours or at high heat for 4 hours.

4. Then remove the roast from the Crockpot and set to a large bowl. Using two forks, shred the meat then toss with the juices from the Crockpot.

5. Serve the roast warm on toast.

Nutritional Information per Serving: Calories 327.9, Fat 25.6g, Carbs 1.8g, Protein 22.9g

Freestyle Swedish Meatballs

Points: 6

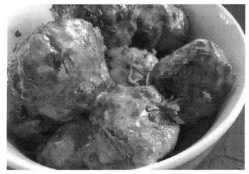

Serves 4

Ingredients

1 tablespoon Dijon mustard

1 tablespoon Worcestershire sauce

1 ½ cups heavy (whipping) cream

1 ½ cups chicken broth

4 tablespoon salted butter

1/4 teaspoon allspice

1/2 teaspoon ground nutmeg

1/4 cup diced onions

1 tablespoon water

1 large egg

1 cup mild Cheddar cheese, shredded

2 lbs. ground meatloaf blend

Directions

1. Preheat your oven to 400 degrees F. Meanwhile, set a slow cooker to the low setting.

2. Using parchment paper, line a large baking pan and set aside.

3. Mix all together, nutmeg, water, onion, egg, cheddar cheese and ground meat.

4. Roll the mixture in 1-and-a-half inch meatballs and layer them onto the baking pan.

5. Bake the meatballs for around 20 minutes. Alternatively, wait until the thermometer reads 140 degrees F.

6. As the meat cooks, heat butter in a small skillet over medium heat along with chicken broth and heavy cream.

7. As soon as it starts to simmer, lower the heat to low and simmer for another 20 minutes while stirring frequently.

8. Once the sauce reduces in half, add in Worcestershire sauce and the mustard. Then transfer the sauce in a slow cooker along with the meatballs.

9. Cook the mixture for 2 hours on low for the meatballs to marinate.

10. Stir after 30 minutes and serve not beyond 2 hours of cooking.

Nutritional Information per Serving: Calories 773, Carbs 3g, Fat 50g, Protein 74g

Tasty Crock Pot Chicken

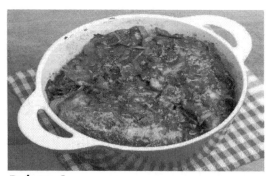

Points: 6
Serves 4
Directions

1 teaspoon white pepper

1/2 teaspoon garlic powder

1/2 teaspoon black pepper

1 teaspoon onion powder

1 teaspoon thyme

1 teaspoon cayenne pepper

2 teaspoons paprika

1 cup chopped onion (optional)

1 large roasting chicken

2 teaspoons salt

Directions

1. Combine the spices in a small bowl.

2. Prepare the chicken by removing any giblets, and then clean the meat.

3. Rub the spice onto the meat and put into a re-sealable plastic bag. Keep under refrigeration preferably overnight.

4. Once ready, place chopped onion into the bottom of slow cooker and cook on low heat for 4-8 hours.

Nutritional Information per Serving: Calories 248, Fat 16g, Carbs 5g, Protein 20g

Slow Cooked Mushroom Stroganoff

Points: 5

Serves 4

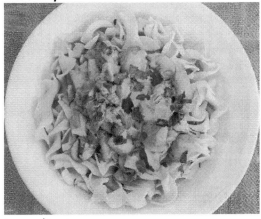

Ingredients

1 cup of spinach

4 Oz cream cheese

1/2 teaspoons paprika

1/2 teaspoon black pepper

1 tablespoon Worcestershire sauce

1 1/2 tablespoons tomato paste

4 oz. sour cream

1 1/2 cups vegetable broth

2 cloves of garlic; minced

1/2 yellow medium onion; diced

4 oz. cremini mushrooms, quartered

8 oz. white mushrooms, quartered

1/2 tablespoon butter

Directions

1. Melt butter in a large pan, and cook the mushroom and onion gently for 5 to 10 minutes, until slightly softened.

2. Transfer to the slow cooker and then stir in the sauce, stock, paprika and garlic.

3. Now cook for 3 or 4 hours on high. Add the chopped parsley and sour cream when cooked, and stir to mix.

4. Once done, serve with rice or pasta.

Nutritional Information per Serving: Calories 207.8, Fat 17.4g, Carbs 8.7g, Protein 7g

Buffalo Chicken Meatballs

Points: 4

Serves 3 (3 meatballs per person)

 Ingredients

1 egg

1/4 cup Parmesan cheese

1/8 teaspoon cayenne pepper

1/8 teaspoon pepper

1/2 teaspoon salt, divided

7 ounces lean chicken or turkey, ground

1 slice sandwich bread

2 tablespoon coconut milk

For Sauce

Dash teaspoon kosher or sea salt

1/4 teaspoon black pepper

1/8 teaspoon cayenne pepper

1/2 teaspoon paprika

1/2 teaspoon chili powder

1/4 cup honey or coconut sugar

1/2 (4 ounce) can diced green chiles

1/2 cup hot sauce

1 clove garlic, minced

1/2 small green onions, diced

1 teaspoon olive oil

Directions

1. First, preheat your oven to 450 degrees F and then line a baking sheet with aluminum foil.

2. Then soak the bread in milk inside a small bowl. In a separate bowl, combine together the meat, egg, salt and the soaked bread. Combine well to create a compact mixture.

3. Obtain a tablespoon of meat and roll it in your palms to create the meatballs, put them in the baking sheet and cook for around 6 minutes.

4. To make the sauce, heat olive oil on medium-low heat then add in garlic and onions. Sauté until the onions become translucent.

5. To a bowl, add in garlic, onions and other ingredients. Whisk until smooth.

6. Now add sufficient meatballs to cover the bottom of the Crockpot, and then pour on half of the sauce.

7. Add in the rest of the meatballs and the remaining sauce. Cover and cook for 2-4 hours on low, or until the balls are well cooked.

Nutritional Information per Serving: Calories: 274, Carbs: 21g, Fat: 11g, Protein: 18g

Greek Chicken & Vegetable Ragout

Points: 4

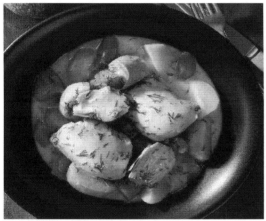

Serves 2 (1⅓ cups)

Ingredients

Pepper, freshly ground

1/3 cup chopped fresh dill

1/3 cup lemon juice

2 large egg yolks

1 large egg

1 15-ounce can artichoke hearts, rinsed

¾ teaspoon salt

4 cloves garlic, minced

1/3 cup dry white wine

1 14-ounce can chicken broth, reduced-sodium

2 pounds boneless, skinless chicken thighs, trimmed

1 pound rutabagas, 1¼-inch-wide wedges

3 cups baby carrots

Directions

1. Spread the rutabagas and the carrots over the slow cooker. Then arrange the chicken over them.

2. Over medium-high heat, bring salt, garlic, wine and broth to simmer in a medium saucepan.

3. Pour the broth mixture over the vegetables and chicken and cover the cooker. Cook for about 4 to 4½ hours on low or 2½ to 3 hours on high.

4. As soon as the veggies are tender and the chicken is cooked through, add artichokes, cover and cook for 5 minutes on High heat.

5. Meanwhile, in a medium bowl, whisk lemon juice, egg yolks and egg until well incorporated.

6. Using a slotted spoon, move the veggies and chicken to a serving boil. Cover to remain warm.

7. At this point, ladle ½ cup of the cooling liquid into the lemon mixture and whisk until smooth. Whisk the mixture into the liquid that remained in the Crockpot.

8. Cover and cook for about 15-20 minutes while whisking occasionally. Remove from heat after the sauce is slightly thickened and has reached a temperature of 160 degrees F.

9. Stir in pepper and dill, and now pour the sauce over the veggies and chicken.

Nutritional Information per Serving: Calories 326, Carbs 23g, Fat 10g, Protein 29g

Wine & Tomato Braised Chicken

Points: 5

Serves 4

Ingredients

1 ½ tablespoons fresh parsley, finely chopped

4 bone-in chicken thighs, skin removed, trimmed

Salt

11.2 ounce whole tomatoes, chopped

6 tablespoons dry white wine

1/2 bay leaf

1/2 teaspoon pepper, freshly ground

1/2 teaspoon fennel seeds

1/2 teaspoon dried thyme

1 1/2 cloves garlic, minced

1/2 large onion, thinly sliced

1½-2 slices of bacon

Direction

1. In a large skillet over medium heat, cook the bacon for about 4 minutes. Once crisp, move to a paper towel, drain and set aside to cool. Crumble.

2. Drain the fat from the pan and reserve 2 tablespoons. Then add the onion and cook for 3-6 minutes over medium heat.

3. Once softened, add in bay leaf, fennel seeds thyme, garlic and pepper. Cook for a minute while stirring.

4. Then add in wine, boil for about 2 minutes while scraping up the browned bits. Now add in tomatoes along with the juice. Add salt and stir to mix.

5. Put the chicken thighs into a Crockpot, and then sprinkle the bacon over the chicken. Pour the wine and tomato mixture and cover the slow cooker.

6. Cook for around 6 hours on low or 3 hours on high or until the chicken is tender. Open the cooker, remove the bay leaf and serve with parsley.

<u>*Enchilada Chicken Stew*</u>

Points: 6
Serves: 4

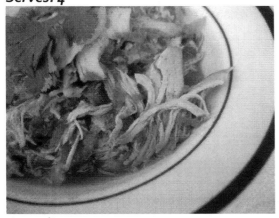

Ingredients

2 teaspoons oregano, dried
1 tablespoon chili powder
1 tablespoon cumin
3 garlic cloves, minced
7 oz.-can tomato sauce
1 (14 oz.) can of diced tomatoes
2 tablespoons coconut oil
1 (4 oz.) can of green chiles, chopped
1 (4 oz.) can of chopped jalapenos
1 green bell pepper, chopped
1 yellow onion, chopped
2 lbs. chicken breasts
Avocado
Bundle of cilantro
Salt and pepper

Directions

1. Add chicken breasts in the slow cooker followed by all other ingredients save for the avocado and cilantro.
2. Now cook in the Crockpot on high heat setting for 6-8 hours or low for 8-10 hours.
3. Use tongs to pick the chicken and then shred it alongside other ingredients.
4. To serve, top with avocado and cilantro.

Nutritional Information per Serving: Calories 373.5, Fat 11.8g, Carbs 14.1g, Protein 51.5g

Italian Beef for Sandwiches

Points: 7
Serves 4

Ingredients

2 pound rump roast
0.3 oz. dry Italian-style salad dressing mix
1/2 bay leaf
1/2 teaspoon garlic powder
1/2 teaspoon dried parsley
1/2 teaspoon onion salt
1/4 teaspoon of basil, dried
1/4 teaspoon of oregano, dried
1/2 teaspoon of black pepper, ground
1/2 teaspoon salt
1 1/4 cups water

Directions

1. In a saucepan, combine together salad dressing mix, bay leaf, garlic powder, parsley, onion salt, basil, oregano, black pepper and salt.
2. Stir the mixture well and bring to a boil.
3. Now put the roast to a Crockpot and season with the dressing mix.
4. Cover and cook on high heat for 4-5 hours or low heat settings for 10 to 12 hours.
5. Once ready, discard the bay leaf then use forks to shred the meat. Serve.

Nutritional Information per Serving: Calories: 318, Fat: 15.8g, Carbs: 1.6g, Protein: 39.4g

Pork Chops with Cream of Mushroom

Points: 6
Serves: 4

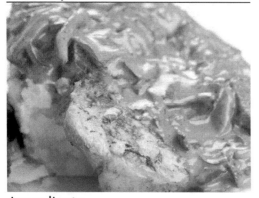

Ingredients
1 cup of water
1 can cream of chicken soup
1 can cream of mushroom soup
4 thick boneless pork chops

Directions

Directions
1. First brown the pork chops in a frying pan and set aside.
2. To a slow cooker or crockpot, add a can of cream of mushroom soup.
3. Then add in the browned pork chops and top with a can of cream of chicken soup.
4. Cook the contents on high for 5 to 6 hours or low heat for 7 to 8 hours.
5. Serve a chop each while top with a ¼ of the gravy.
Nutritional Information per Serving: Calories 284.6, Fat 16.2g, Carbs 10.6g, Protein 23.2g

Meatballs with Ranch-Buffalo Sauce

Serves: 10, Cooking Time: 2 hours, Preparation Time: 5 minutes
Ingredients:
- 1 packet Hidden Valley Ranch dressing dry mix
- 1 bottle Frank's red-hot wings buffalo sauce
- 1 bag frozen Rosina Italian style Meat balls

Instructions:
1. Grease sides and bottom of Slow Cooker with cooking spray.
2. Mix dressing mix and buffalo sauce in slow cooker.
3. Add meat balls and evenly spread on bottom of pot.
4. Cover and cook on high for two hours.
5. Serve and enjoy.

Nutrition information:

Calories per serving: 219; Carbohydrates: 31.21g; Protein: 5.98g; Fat: 7.88g; Sugar: 25.43g; Sodium: 791mg; Fiber: 1.2g

Moroccan Chicken in Slow Cooker

Points: 5
Serves: 4
Cooking Time: hours minutes
Preparation Time: minutes
Ingredients:
- ½ teaspoon salt
- 2 cups water
- 1 medium onion, chopped coarsely
- 8 pieces chicken thighs, skinless
- ½ cup prunes
- 1 ¼ teaspoons curry powder
- ½ teaspoon ground cinnamon

Instructions:
1. In slow cooker, mix well salt, water, curry powder, and cinnamon.
2. Add prunes and onions.
3. Place chicken in a single layer in slow cooker, if possible.
4. Cover and cook for 4 hours on high settings.

Nutrition information:

Calories per serving: 958; Carbohydrates: 55.73g; Protein: 50.65g; Fat: 59.96g; Sugar: 1.19g; Sodium: 2465mg; Fiber: 1g

Meatballs with Pineapple-Soy Sauce

Points: 7
Serves: 10
Cooking Time: 2 hours
Preparation Time: 5 minutes
Ingredients:
- 1 20-ounce can pineapple tidbits, with juice
- 1 bag fully cooked frozen Rosina Italian Meatballs
- 1 stalk sliced green onions
- ¼ teaspoons sesame seeds
- ¼ cup soy sauce

Instructions:
1. Mix well pineapple, juice, and soy sauce.
2. Add meatballs and spread in a single layer on bottom of slow cooker.
3. Cover and cook on high for 2 hours.
4. To serve, sprinkle sesame seeds and green onions on top.

Nutrition information:

Calories per serving: 145; Carbohydrates: 11.11g; Protein: 6.22g; Fat: 8.75g; Sugar: 9.02g; Sodium: 325mg; Fiber: 1g

Delicious Chicken BBQ Ranch

Serves: 4, Cooking Time: 4 hours 30 minutes, Preparation Time: 20 minutes
Ingredients:
- 4 boneless skinless chicken breasts, thawed
- 1 Hidden Valley Ranch seasoning mix packet
- 1-pound bacon
- 1 tablespoon barbecue powder
- 1 cup water

Instructions:
1. In slow cooker, place chicken and water. Cover and cook on high for 4 hours.
2. On nonstick skillet, place on medium high fire and cook bacon until crisped, around 3 minutes per side. Remove from pan and crumble.
3. In medium bowl, mix well ranch seasoning, and barbecue powder.
4. Once chicken is done cooking, remove from pot and chop or shred.
5. Return chicken to pot and pour in seasoning mixture and mix well.
6. Cover and cook for another 30 minutes.

Nutrition information:

Calories per serving: 642; Carbohydrates: 8.43g; Protein: 65.35g; Fat: 39.68g; Sugar: 0.23g; Sodium: 1927mg; Fiber: 3.2g

Chicken Enchilada Style

Points: 5, Serves: 4, Cooking Time: 3 hours 30 minutes, Preparation Time: 5 minutes

Ingredients:

- 1 cup Mexican cheese, shredded
- 1 can mild green chilies, drained
- 2 teaspoons garlic salt
- 1 10-ounce can La Victoria mild red enchilada sauce
- 4 boneless, skinless chicken breasts, thawed

Instructions:

1. Place chicken in slow cooker and season with garlic salt. Cover and cook on high settings for 3 hours.
2. Meanwhile, in a bowl mix well green chilies and enchilada sauce.
3. Once chicken is done cooking, discard sauce inside slow cooker.
4. Pour enchilada sauce over chicken and then sprinkle cheese on top.
5. Cover and cook for another 30 minutes.

Nutrition information:

Calories per serving: 964; Carbohydrates: 43.18g; Protein: 88.14g; Fat: 47.41g; Sugar: 2.55g; Sodium: 2056mg; Fiber: 1.8g

Pork Loin with Cherry-Balsamic Sauce

Points: 7, Serves: 6, Cooking Time: 6 hours 12 minutes, Preparation Time: 20 minutes

Ingredients:

- ½ teaspoon pepper
- 1 teaspoon salt
- 1 tablespoon canola oil
- 1 boneless pork loin roast, 3-pounds
- 1/3 cup balsamic vinegar
- ½ cup dried cherries

Instructions:

1. Season roast with salt and pepper.
2. On a large pan on medium high fire, heat oil.
3. Brow roast on all sides, around 3 minutes per side.
4. Transfer roast into slow cooker.
5. Add all remaining ingredient sin pot.
6. Cover and cook on low for 6 hours.

Nutrition information:

Calories per serving: 525; Carbohydrates: 4.56g; Protein: 82.21g; Fat: 17.21g; Sugar: 3.83g; Sodium: 572mg; Fiber: 0.3g

Crock Pot Pork in Ranch Sauce

Points: 5, Serves: 6, Cooking Time: 4 hours, Preparation Time: 20 minutes

Ingredients:
- ¼ cup water
- 1 cup milk
- 1 envelope ranch salad dressing mix
- 2 cans 10.75-ounce each, condensed cream of chicken soup
- 6 boneless pork loin chops, 6-ounces each

Instructions:
1. Mix all ingredients in slow cooker.
2. Cover and cook on low settings for 4 hours.

Nutrition information:

Calories per serving: 324; Carbohydrates: 10.62g; Protein: 46.33g; Fat: 9.41g; Sugar: 2.61g; Sodium: 494mg; Fiber: 1g

Pork Chops with Cranberry Sauce

Points: 4, Serves: 6, Cooking Time: 6 hours, Preparation Time: 10 minutes

Ingredients:
- Salt and pepper to taste
- 6-pieces bone-in pork loin chops
- 1 14-ounce can whole-berry cranberry sauce, unsweetened
- 1 2/3-cups unsweetened applesauce

Instructions:
1. Mix well cranberry sauce and apple sauce in slow cooker.
2. Season chops generously with salt and pepper.
3. Place chops on topo of sauce.
4. Cover and cook on low for 6 hours.

Nutrition information:

Calories per serving: 460; Carbohydrates: 34.1g; Protein: 40.61g; Fat: 17.55g; Sugar: 31.83g; Sodium: 107mg; Fiber: 1.5g

Pizzaiola Steak Slow Cooker

Points: 7, Serves: 4, Cooking Time: 8 hours, Preparation Time: 5 minutes

Ingredients:
- ¼ cup water
- 2-pounds London broil
- 1 medium sliced onion
- 1 red, orange, or yellow sweet sliced bell pepper
- Half a jar of pasta sauce

Instructions:
1. In slow cooker, mix well water and pasta sauce.
2. Place London broil and top with bell pepper and onion.
3. Cover and cook on low for 8 hours.

Nutrition information:

Chicken Breasts with Onions and Mushrooms

Points: 6
Serves 4

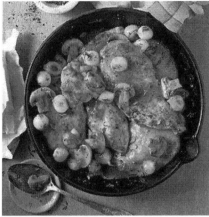

Ingredients
Salt and Pepper
Thyme
1 cup chicken broth
2 large bone-in split chicken breasts
1 cup sliced mushrooms
1 sliced onions

Directions
1. First line the bottom of the crockpot with onions, and then put the chicken breast on top.
2. Top the chicken meat with more onions and pour chicken broth around the edge of the crockpot.
3. Now add in thyme, pepper and salt and cook for 6 to 8 hour on low heat setting.

Nutritional Information per Serving: Calories 235.1, Fat 12.5 g, Carbs 18.3g, Protein 12.8 g

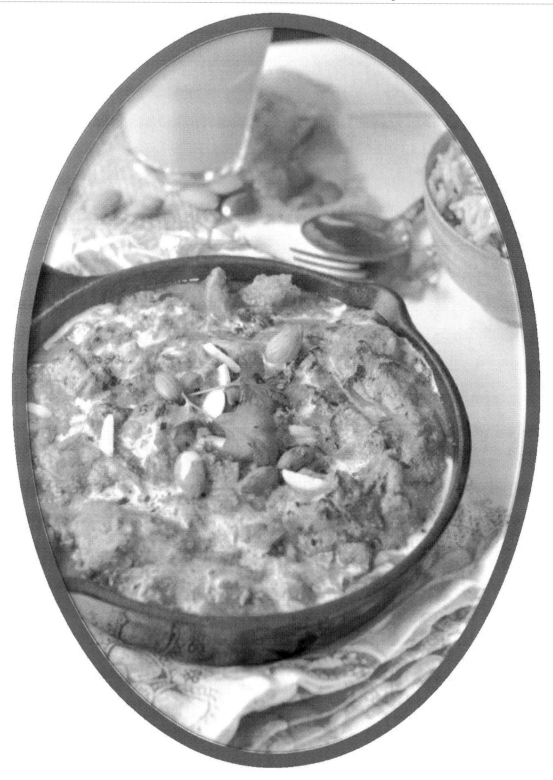

Easy Meatball Crock Pot

Points: 6

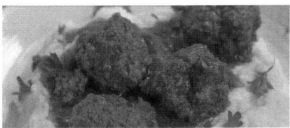

Serves: 3

Ingredients

For the meatballs:

1 heaping tablespoon tomato paste

1 cup bone broth

Sea salt and pepper

1/2 teaspoon paprika

1/2 tablespoon cumin

1 lb. ground beef

Small handful fresh parsley, diced

For the cauliflower:

Sea salt

2 tablespoons butter or ghee

1/2 large head a cauliflower

Pepper

Directions:

1. Put the meat in a bowl along with pepper, salt, paprika and cumin. Mix well to blend.

2. Make the meat into one-inch meatballs and put the balls at the bottom of a crockpot.

3. Then mix the paste and the broth in a bowl and pour over the meatballs. Set the crockpot on high and cook for about 2 hours.

4. Once the meatballs are cooked through, chop the cauliflower into florets and then steam them until well cooked.

5. Now discard the water and add in salt, butter and pepper. Blend the mixture using an immersion blender until smooth.

6. Put the cauliflower mash onto serving plate, top with meatballs and enough amount of sauce on top.

7. Garnish with parsley and enjoy.

Nutritional Information per Serving: Calories: 413, Protein: 46.7g, Fat: 17.4g, Carbs: 2.5g

Chicken Hearts Stroganoff

Points: 5
Serves 3

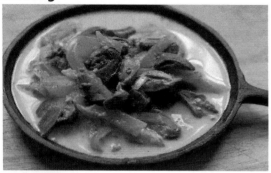

Ingredients

7 tablespoons full fat Greek yogurt

2 tablespoons heavy cream or coconut milk

1/2 cup chicken stock

1/4 tablespoon cayenne pepper

1/4 tablespoon paprika

½ teaspoon pepper

½ teaspoon salt

½ tablespoon Dijon mustard

2 cloves garlic, minced

1 lb. chicken hearts, cut into thirds

1/2 lb. (8 ounce) whole mushrooms, sliced

½ onion, thinly sliced

Directions

1. Add mushrooms and onions to the slow cooker then top with chicken hearts. The meat should not touch the sides.

2. Add in species, garlic and mustard then pour in chicken stock.

3. Cover the crockpot and cook for 6 hours on low heat. Then turn off the heat, let cool for 5 minutes and then stir in yoghurt and cream.

4. Let cool for about 5 minutes before serving. If need be, you can use other types of thickeners such as sour cream or Crème fraiche. Serve with steamed veggies.

Nutritional Information per Serving: Calories 249.4, Fat6.3g, Carbs 9.7g, Protein 38.7g

Poached Salmon in Slow Cooker

Points: 4, Serves: 4, Cooking Time: 60 minutes, Preparation Time: 5 minutes
Ingredients:

●1 cup water

●½ teaspoon salt

●4 (6-ounce) salmon fillets

●1 dill sprig

●1 sliced lemon

- 1 yellow onion sliced

Instructions:

1. Make a pouch out of foil. Spray with cooking spray to prevent salmon from sticking on foil.
2. Place salmon fillet in foil.
3. Season with salt.
4. Add dill and onion.
5. Securely seal foil to make a bag.
6. Place in slow cooker and add water.
7. Cover and cook for an hour on high.

Nutrition information:

Calories per serving: 331; Carbohydrates: 2.79g; Protein: 38.31g; Fat: 17.53g; Sugar: 1.32g; Sodium: 1250mg; Fiber: 0.4g

Crockpot Smoky Baby Back Ribs

Points: 7, Serves: 4, Cooking Time: 9 hours, Preparation Time: 5 minutes

Ingredients:

- 1 ½ teaspoon barbecue sauce
- 1 ½ teaspoon hoisin sauce
- ½ teaspoon smoked paprika
- 2 ½ pounds baby back ribs
- 1 cup water

Instructions:

1. Evenly season ribs with barbecue sauce, hoisin sauce, and smoked paprika.
2. Grease slow cooker with cooking spray and add seasoned ribs.
3. Add water, cover and cook on low settings for 9 hours.

Nutrition information:

Calories per serving: 723; Carbohydrates: 3.74g; Protein: 53.2g; Fat: 55.01g; Sugar: 1.3g; Sodium: 228mg; Fiber: 0.2g

Beef Italian Sandwiches

Points: 6, Serves: 6, Cooking Time: 9 hours, Preparation Time: 15 minutes

Ingredients:

- Provolone cheese slices
- 14.5-ounce can beef broth
- 8-ounces giardiniera drained (Chicago-style Italian sandwich mix)
- 3-pounds chuck roast fat trimmed and cut into large pieces
- 6 large lettuce

Instructions:

1. In slow cooker add beef broth, sandwich mix, and chuck roast.
2. Cook on low for 9 hours or on high for 5 hours.
3. Remove from pot and with two forks shred beef.
4. To make a sandwich, add warm shredded beef in one lettuce leaf and top with cheese.

Nutrition information:

Calories per serving: 538; Carbs: 3.86g; Protein: 48.63g; Fat: 36.42g; Sugar: 1.9g; Sodium: 707mg; Fiber: 1.4g

Lettuce Taco Carnitas

Points: 5, Serves: 12, Cooking Time: 6 hours, Preparation Time: 15 minutes

Ingredients:

- 2 cups shredded Colby-Monterey jack cheese
- 1 can (10-ounces) green chilies and diced tomatoes, undrained
- 1 envelope taco seasoning
- 1 boneless pork shoulder butt roast (4-pounds)
- Lettuce leaves

Instructions:

1. In slow cooker, mix well diced tomatoes, taco seasoning, and pork.
2. Cover and cook for 9 hours on low setting.
3. Once tender, remove from pot and shred with two forks.
4. To serve, add a good amount of shredded pork into center of one lettuce leaf. Top it with cheese, roll, and enjoy.

Nutrition information:

Calories per serving: 214; Carbohydrates: 1.68g; Protein: 28.53g; Fat: 10.39g; Sugar: 0.22g; Sodium: 340mg; Fiber: 0.1g

Chicken Adobo Filipino Style

Points: 6, Serves: 6, Cooking Time: 6 hours, Preparation Time: 15 minutes

Ingredients:

- 1 cup water
- ¼ cup vinegar
- 6 skinless, boneless chicken breast halves (6-ounces each), cut into 1-inch cubes
- 3 garlic cloves
- 1 bay leaf
- ¼ cup soy sauce

Instructions:

1. Mix all ingredients in pot.
2. Cover and cook on low for 6 hours.
3. Best served with a side of rice.

Nutrition information:

Calories per serving: 240; Carbohydrates: 3.46g; Protein: 39.15g; Fat: 6.41g; Sugar: 2.1g; Sodium: 239mg; Fiber: 0.3g

Beans with Shredded Pork

Points: 5, Serves: 12, Cooking Time: 5 hours, Preparation Time: 20 minutes

Ingredients:

- 1 jar (24-ounces) picante sauce
- 2 cans (15-ounces each) black beans drained and rinsed
- 3-pounds pork tenderloin, cut into 3-inch lengths

Instructions:

1. In slow cooker, mix pork and picante sauce.

2. Cover and cook for 4 hours on high.
3. Remove pork, shred and return to pot.
4. Add black beans and continue cooking for another hour.

Nutrition information:

Calories per serving: 239; Carbs: 11.25g; Protein: 32.1g; Fat: 4.68g; Sugar: 4.78g; Sodium: 994mg; Fiber: 5.2g

Freestyle Slow-Cooker Beef & Broccoli

Points: 6

Serves 4

Ingredients

1 red bell pepper

1 head broccoli

1/2 teaspoon salt

1/4 - 1/2 teaspoon red pepper flakes

3 garlic cloves, minced

1 teaspoon freshly grated ginger

3 tablespoon your sweetener

1 cup beef broth

2/3 cup liquid aminos

2 lbs. flank steak

1 teaspoon sesame seeds, optional

Directions

1. Begin by setting the slow cooker to the low setting. Then proceed to slice a flank steak into chunks.

2. Once hot, add the steak, salt, pepper, garlic, sweetener, beef broth and coconut aminos to the crockpot.

3. Cook the ingredients for about 5 to 6 hours. Prepare bell pepper and broccoli. Simply slice the bell pepper into 1 inch pieces and chop the broccoli to florets.

4. Once cooked, stir the steak then add in red pepper and chopped broccoli. Cook for about 1 hour until crisp, and then toss the mixture together.

5. At this point, sprinkle with sesame and serve garnished with sesame seeds if you like it. You can also serve over cauliflower rice.

6. If need be, thicken the sauce using arrowroot thickener. Just combine 2 tablespoons of water with a tablespoon of arrowroot thickener and add to the steak mixture once cooked through. Add enough of it until you achieve desired consistency.

Nutritional Information per Serving: Calories 430, Fat 19g, Carbs 4g, Protein 54g

Chocolate Chicken Mole

Points: 7
Serves: 3

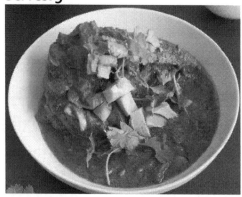

Ingredients

1/4 teaspoon chili powder

1/4 teaspoon cinnamon power, ground

½ teaspoon cumin powder

½ teaspoon sea salt

1. 25 oz. (35.4 g) dark chocolate 70% or above

2 tablespoons creamy almond butter

2 ½ dried New Mexico chili peppers rehydrated and chopped

3-4 whole tomatoes peeled, seeded and chopped

2 cloves garlic crushed or minced

½ medium onion chopped

1 tablespoon ghee

Sea salt

Black pepper to taste

1 lb. chicken pieces bone in breasts and legs, without skin

Cilantro, avocado and jalapeno, chopped

Directions

1. Season the chicken with salt and pepper and set aside. Put a pan over medium heat on a skillet then add in ghee.

2. Once melted, add in chicken and brown it on both sides. If the chicken is large, you can do it in batches.

3. Now transfer the chicken to a crockpot. Then add in onion to the pan with chicken then sauté until golden. Add in garlic and sauté for about a minute or so.

4. Once done, move the garlic and onion to the crockpot along with spices, salt, dark chocolate, almond butter, chili peppers and tomatoes.

5. Cook until the chicken is tender and can easily pull about, or for about 6 to 8 hours

6. To serve, top with jalapeno, cilantro and avocado.

Nutritional Information per Serving: Calories 402.1, Fat 20.4g, Carbs 20.6g, Protein 37.0g

New Mexico Carne Adovada

Points: 4
Serves 4

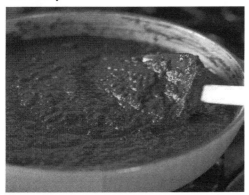

Ingredients

2 teaspoons apple cider vinegar

1 teaspoon kosher salt, or to taste

1 teaspoon ground coriander

1 teaspoon ground cumin

2 teaspoons dried Mexican oregano

6 cloves garlic, chopped

1 onion, chopped

2 cups chicken or beef stock

6 -8 ounces dried New Mexican chiles, rinsed

3 pounds pork shoulder, cut into 1 inch cubes

Directions

1. Discard the seeds from peppers and then break them into smaller pieces. You can also roast them in your oven for 5 to 10 minutes at 300 degrees F if not dry enough to break.

2. Then put the chile pieces in a large pot along with the rest of the ingredients, save from the pork. Cover and simmer the mixture for 30-60 minutes under low heat setting.

3. Once cooked well, remove from heat then let cool for a few minutes. Then using a hand blender or food processor, puree the mixture in batches.

4. Use a wire sauce to strain the red chile sauce to obtain a smoother sauce. Add in water or broth if needed to achieve the preferred thickness.

5. At this point, put the pork meat in a deep baking dish and cover with the sauce. Keep it refrigerated for 1 to 2 days to marinate. Remember to stir frequently.

6. Then bring the mixture back to room temperature and cook in a slow cooker for 4 to 6 hours on low heat.

7. Serve as soon as the pork is fork tender and the sauce is cooked down. Serve warm or hot with sliced tomatoes, tortillas, cornbread, avocado or cooling salad.

Nutritional Information per Serving: Calories 120.2, Fat 5.3g, Carb 11.3g, Protein 8.0g

Beef Chuck Pot Roast

Points: 8
Serves: 2-3

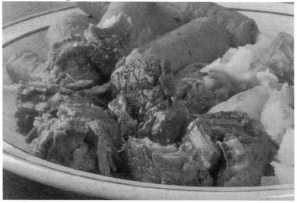

Ingredients
1/4 can cream of celery soup or cream of mushroom soup
1/4 packet onion soup dry mix
1 lb. beef for roasting

Directions
1. Begin by stabbing the meat in a few places using a fork or knife, and place in crock-pot with the side with the fatty side facing up.
2. Add the dry onion soup on top and on sides followed with the can of mushroom or celery soup over the roast.
3. Spread it on top a little and now cover the slow cooker and turn it on!
4. At this point, cook for 3 hours on high or 5 hours set on low heat setting.
5. If need be, set the slow cooker on low and allow the roast in- in the morning to prepare for an evening meal.

Nutritional Information per Serving: Calories 280, Carbs 2.5g, Fat 13.2g, Proteins 35.5g

Crockpot Turkey Breast

Points: 6
Serves: 4

Ingredients
6 tablespoons butter separated
1 cup chicken broth
12-15 baby carrots
2 yellow onions
5 stalks celery
1 (5-6 pounds) bone-in turkey breast, thawed

Seasonings
1/4 teaspoon dried sage
1/4 teaspoon dried parsley
1 teaspoon Italian seasoning

1/2 teaspoon pepper

1 teaspoon paprika

1 teaspoon seasoned salt

1 tablespoon dried garlic, minced

1/4 teaspoon dried thyme, optional

Directions

1. Thaw the turkey inside the fridge for around 1-2 days. Then coat your slow cooker with non-stick spray.

2. Add celery to the bottom of the Crockpot, cut a yellow onion into large chunks and add to the cooker. Add in baby carrots along with chicken broth.

3. Put the turkey breast on the veggies, breast side down. Then cut the onion in half and put it inside the turkey along with 4 tablespoons butter.

4. Mix together all the seasonings in a bowl, and rub on the meat. If the breast has skin on, also rub the seasonings under the skin.

5. Meanwhile, melt about 2 tablespoons of butter and brush all over the seasoned breast using a pastry brush.

6. Cover the slow cooker and cook the contents on high for 1 hour. Lower the heat and now cook for 5-7 hours or until the turkey is tender. Check if the internal temperature has reached 165 degrees.

7. Once done, remove the turkey breast from the slow cooker, and break it up. Just remove the wishbone and other bones. Pick the large pieces of the turkey and slice them.

Nutritional Information per Serving: 330 Calories, Carbs 3.7g, Fat 17.9g, Protein 38g

Coffee- Braised Brisket

Points: 7

Servings: 4

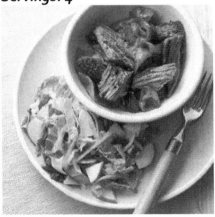

Ingredients

1/2 tablespoon of balsamic vinegar

4 cup of strong brewed coffee

1 large sliced onion

1/2 (3-pound) boneless beef brisket

1/2 teaspoon of salt

1/2 teaspoon of ground black pepper

1/2 teaspoon of garlic powder

1/2 tablespoon of paprika

1/2 tablespoon of ground coffee

1 tablespoons of coconut sugar

Directions

1. Mix together brown sugar, paprika, garlic powder, pepper, salt and ground coffee.

2. Then trim the fat from brisket and rub the mixture over all the surfaces of the brisket. If need be, cut the meat such that it fits into a 4 –quart slow cooker.

3. Put the meat in the Crock Pot and put the onions over a brisket. Then mix vinegar and coffee and pour over onions.

4. Cover and now cook on low-heat for 10 hours or on high heat setting for 5 hours.

5. Once done cooking, move the meat to a cutting board and slice it across the grain.

6. Then remove the onions with slotted spoon from the cooking liquid. Serve the onion mixture with the meat.

Nutritional Information per Serving: Calories 229, Proteins 32g, Carbs 8g, Fat 8g

Slow Cooker Chicken Stroganoff

Points: 7

Servings: 4

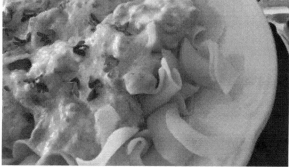

Ingredients

1 (10.75 ounce) can-condensed cream, chicken soup

1 (8 ounce) package of cream cheese

1 (7 ounce) package of dry Italian style salad dressing mixture

1/8 cup of margarine

4 skinless, boneless chicken breasts halves (cubed)

Directions

1. Place the chicken, dressing and margarine into a Crock Pot and mix together.

2. Cook on low heat for 6 hours.

3. Then add in the cream cheese, the soup and combine together.

4. Finally cook on high heat for an extra ½ hour or until it is warm and heated through.

Nutritional Information per Serving: Calories 456, Proteins 33.4g, Fat 31g, Carbs 9.5 G

Crockpot Creamy Salsa Chicken

Points: 7
Servings: 4

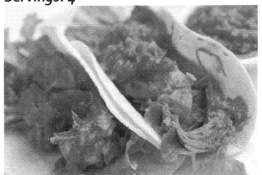

Ingredients
1/2 jar salsa (16 ounce)
1/2 can of cream mushroom soup
3 large boneless chicken breasts

Directions
1. Put the chicken breasts into the bottom of a slow cooker; then combine the cans of salsa and soup.
2. Pour over the chicken breasts and set the slow cooker on low heat.
3. Cook for at least 4 hours and then stir the chicken around using a fork to shred it.
4. In case it does not shred, cook further for about 30 minutes.
5. You can serve with flour tortilla or just as it is. You may also top with onion, avocado or cheese if desired.

Nutritional Information per Serving: Calories 254.6, Protein 40.8g, Carbs 5.3g, Fat 6.6g

Slow Cooker Gumbo

Points: 6
Serves 3

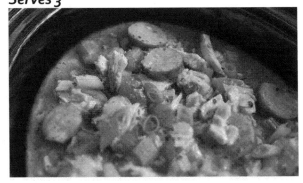

Ingredients
1/4 teaspoon dried basil
½ teaspoon paprika
¼ teaspoon oregano
¼ teaspoon mustard powder

¼ teaspoon cayenne pepper

¼ teaspoon onion powder

¼ teaspoon pepper

1/2 teaspoon kosher salt

½ bay leaf

1 1/2 cups low-sodium chicken broth

½ green bell pepper, chopped

1 clove of garlic, minced

1 cup frozen okra

1 celery stalk, chopped

½ sweet onion, diced

1 turkey andouille sausage links, sliced

1 ½ boneless, skinless chicken breasts

Directions

1. In a Crockpot, add all the ingredients and then cook at high for 3-4 hours or low at 6-8 hours.

2. Once ready, serve over cauliflower rice and enjoy.

Nutritional Information per Serving: Calories: 230, Carbs: 11g, Fat: 6g, Protein: 34g

Slow Cooker Pork Loin

Points: 8

Serves 4

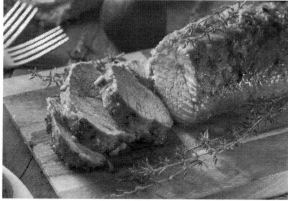

Ingredients

1/4 cup orange juice

1/2 tablespoon curry powder

1/2 teaspoon chicken bouillon granules

1/4 teaspoon ground ginger

1/8 teaspoon ground cinnamon

1/4 teaspoon salt

1/2 small onion, chopped

1/2 clove garlic, minced

1/8 cup raisins

1/8 cup flaked coconut

1 tablespoon cold water

2 pounds boneless pork loin, cut into 1-inch cubes, diced

1 tablespoon arrow root powder

Directions

1. Combine salt, cinnamon, chicken bouillon, curry powder, and orange in a slow cooker.

2. Then proceed to stir in the coconut, raisins, garlic, onion, and apple before placing the pork cubes into the sauce.

3. Next, combine the put the potato starch into water and stir well (use a small bowl) until you cannot see any lumps. Once properly mixed, put everything into a slow cooker.

4. At this point, cover and cook on low until the pork is very tender, let's say for 5 to 6 hours.

Nutritional Information per Serving: Calories 174, Fat 6g, Carbs 8g, Protein 22g

Spicy Crockpot Double Beef Stew

Points: 6

Serves 3

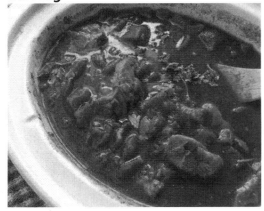

Ingredients

Salt

½ tablespoon Worcestershire sauce

1 teaspoon hot sauce

1/2 cup beef broth

1/2 tablespoon chili mix

1 14.5oz can of chili-ready diced tomatoes

0.75 lbs. (12 ounces) Beef Stew meats

Directions

1. Set the slow cooker to high then add in all the ingredients. Mix to blend.

2. Cook on high heat for 6 hours. Open the lid, break up the meat with a fork and pull apart within the cooking pot.

3. Season with salt and cook another 2 hours on low heat.

Nutritional Information per Serving: Calories 222, Fat 7g, Carbs 11g, Protein 27g

Slow Cooker Balsamic Chicken

Points: 7

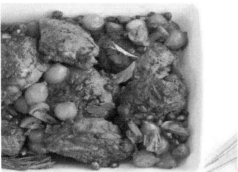

Serves: 4

Ingredients

¼ cup flat leaf parsley leaves

½ cup pomegranate seeds

1 tablespoon butter

Black pepper, freshly ground

Kosher salt

¼ cup coconut sugar

3 tablespoons tomato paste

1 cup chicken stock

¾ cup balsamic vinegar

1 bay leaf

2 stems fresh rosemary

5 garlic cloves, minced

8 ounces white button mushrooms, quartered

1 16 ounce package white pearl onions, frozen

1-2 tablespoons extra virgin olive oil

8-10 boneless, skinless chicken thighs

Directions

1. Season the chicken thigh with pepper and salt.

2. In a large frying pan, heat olive oil over medium heat.

3. Brown the thighs in oil for 5 minutes on each side, in batches. Once golden brown, remove from the pan and set aside.

4. Layer the onions, rosemary, garlic, mushrooms and bay leafs in a bowl of a Crockpot.

5. Add the browned chicken breast to the Crockpot. Mix together balsamic vinegar, brown sugar, tomato paste and chicken stock in a bowl then season with pepper and salt.

6. Pour the mixture over the breast and cook for 3 hours on high. Test for doneness and cook for additional 15-30 minutes if necessary or until the chicken is no longer pink.

7. Move the chicken to a serving dish and cover with foil or lid. Then separate the liquid from the veggies, and add the veggies to the chicken.

8. Add the liquid to a pan and cook over medium high heat. Boil until it has reduced by half, in 5 minutes.

9. Add in butter and whisk until the sauce has thickened and butter melted.

10. Garnish the chicken with parsley and pomegranate. Serve with balsamic sauce.

Nutritional Information per Serving: 280 Calories, Carbs 13.8g, Fat 10.5g, Protein 31.2g

Chicken Slow Cooker Greek Style

Points: 5, Serves: 4, Cooking Time: 4 hours, Preparation Time: 5 minutes

Ingredients:

- ¼ cup feta cheese
- Sliced and pitted Kalamata olives
- 1 bottle (16-ounce) ken's steak house Greek dressing with Feta cheese, olive oil, and black olives
- 4 boneless and skinless thawed chicken breasts

Instructions:

1. Pan Fry chicken for 5 minutes per side. Then chop into bite size pieces and spread evenly in bottom of slow cooker.
2. Add dressing.
3. Cover and cook for 3 hours on high.
4. To serve, sprinkle olives and feta cheese.
5. Enjoy.

Nutrition information:

Calories per serving: 818; Carbohydrates: 3.24g; Protein: 54.44g; Fat: 65.1g; Sugar: 3.22g; Sodium: 204mg; Fiber: 0g

Chicken Salsa in Slow Cooker

Points: 6, Serves: 4, Cooking Time: 5 hours, Preparation Time: 10 minutes

Ingredients:

- 1 cup shredded cheddar cheese
- 8-ounces cream cheese
- 16-ounces salsa
- 4 skinless and boneless thawed chicken breasts
- 1 can corn

Instructions:

1. Chop chicken into ½ inch cubes.
2. Spread chicken evenly on bottom of pot and add salsa.
3. Cover and cook on high for 3 hours.
4. Stir in corn and cream cheese.
5. Cook for another 2 hours.
6. To serve, sprinkle cheese.

Nutrition information:

Calories per serving: 658; Carbs: 31.83g; Protein: 67.76g; Fat: 32.65g; Sugar: 10.42g; Sodium: 1649mg; Fiber: 3.5g

Chicken Country Style

Points: 7
Serves: 4
Cooking Time: 8 hours
Preparation Time: 5 minutes

Ingredients:
- 1/3 teaspoon pepper
- 1 packet dry Lipton's onion soup mix
- 1 can (14.5-ounce) Campbell's chicken gravy
- 4 skinless and boneless chicken breasts

Instructions:
1. Chop chicken into 1-inch cubes and spread evenly on bottom of slow cooker.
2. Add all ingredients and mix well.
3. Cover and cook for 8 hours on low.

Nutrition information:

Calories per serving: 366; Carbohydrates: 6.81g; Protein: 53.7g; Fat: 11.88g; Sugar: 2.09g; Sodium: 591mg; Fiber: 0.1g

Broccoli Chicken Crockpot

Points: 4, Serves: 4, Cooking Time: 3 hours 30 minutes, Preparation Time: 5 minutes

Ingredients:
- ½ cup water
- 1 package frozen chopped broccoli (10-ounces)
- 1 cup shredded sharp cheddar cheese
- ½ cup sour cream
- 1 can Campbell's broccoli cheese soup
- 4 boneless skinless chicken breasts, thawed

Instructions:
1. Chop chicken in ½-inch cubes and spread on bottom of slow cooker.
2. Stir in cheese soup and water.
3. Cover and cook on high for 3 hours.
4. Stir in sour cream, cheese, and chopped broccoli.
5. Continue cooking for another 2 hours.

Nutrition information:

Calories per serving: 511; Carbohydrates: 11.71g; Protein: 63.93g; Fat: 22.11g; Sugar: 2.14g; Sodium: 554mg; Fiber: 3.2g

Whole Barbecue Chicken

Points: 5, Serves: 6, Cooking Time: 4 hours, Preparation Time: 10 minutes

Ingredients:
- ½ cup water
- 1 sliced white onion
- 2 packets McCormick grill mates Tennessee smokehouse barbecue rub
- Whole chicken (5-pounds)

Instructions:

1. Add water in slow cooker.
2. Rub chicken with the barbecue rub, inside and out.
3. Place half of the sliced onion inside the chicken.
4. Place chicken in slow cooker and sprinkle remaining onions.
5. Cover and cook for 4 hours on high.

Nutrition information:

Calories per serving: 194; Carbohydrates: 0.82g; Protein: 33.85g; Fat: 5.14g; Sugar: 0.1g; Sodium: 246mg; Fiber: 0g

One Pot Chicken Chipotle

Points: 6, Serves: 4, Cooking Time: 4 hours, Preparation Time: 10 minutes

Ingredients:

- ½ cup water
- 4 tablespoons McCormick grill mates' chipotle
- Roasted garlic seasoning
- 8 garlic cloves peeled and crushed
- 5-pounds whole chicken

Instructions:

1. Rub chipotle and garlic seasoning all over chicken, inside and out.
2. Place half of the garlic cloves inside the chicken.
3. Place chicken in slow cooker and add water.
4. Sprinkle remaining garlic on chicken and water.
5. Cover and cook on high for 4 hours.

Nutrition information:

Calories per serving: 1226; Carbohydrates: 115.69g; Protein: 100.62g; Fat: 41.4g; Sugar: 20.37g; Sodium: 2080mg; Fiber: 17.3g

Tender Turkey Breast

Points: 7, Serves: 12, Cooking Time: 4 hours, Preparation Time: 10 minutes

Ingredients:

- ¼ teaspoon salt
- ½ cup water
- ½ teaspoon coarsely ground pepper
- 4 peeled garlic cloves
- 4 fresh rosemary sprigs
- 1 bone-in turkey breast (7-pounds)

Instructions:

1. Rub all seasoning on turkey.
2. Place turkey in pot, makes sure that you also add all seasoning in pot.
3. Add water.
4. Cover and cook for 4 hours on high.

Nutrition information:

Calories per serving: 179; Carbohydrates: 0.82g; Protein: 35.77g; Fat: 2.69g; Sugar: 0.38g; Sodium: 166mg; Fiber: 0.1g

Slow Cooked Steak Swiss

Points: 7, Serves: 6, Cooking Time: 8 hours, Preparation Time: 10 minutes

Ingredients:

- ½ teaspoon salt
- ¼ teaspoon pepper
- 2 (8-ounce) cans tomato sauce
- 1 celery rib, cut into ½-inch slices
- 1 medium onion, sliced into ¼-inch pieces
- 1 ½-pounds beef round steak, cut into 6 pieces

Instructions:

1. Add all ingredients in slow cooker.
2. Mix well.
3. Cover and cook for 8 hours on low.
4. Serve and enjoy.

Nutrition information:

Calories per serving: 236; Carbohydrates: 17.28g; Protein: 27.34g; Fat: 4.6g; Sugar: 8.14g; Sodium: 1276mg; Fiber: 4.6g

Cranberry Gravy Brisket

Points: 5, Serves: 7, Cooking Time: 8 hours, Preparation Time: 15 minutes

Ingredients:

- ½ teaspoon salt
- ¼ teaspoon pepper
- 1 tablespoon prepared mustard
- ½ cup chopped onion
- 1 (8-ounce) can tomato sauce
- 1 (14-ounce) whole-berry cranberry sauce
- 1 fresh beef brisket (2 ½-pounds)

Instructions:

1. Chop beef into 1-inch cubes and spread on bottom of slow cooker.
2. Add remaining ingredients into pot.
3. Cover and cook on low for 8 hours.
4. Serve and enjoy.

Nutrition information:

Calories per serving: 264; Carbohydrates: 29.74g; Protein: 24.91g; Fat: 24.41g; Sugar: 25.36g; Sodium: 2613mg; Fiber: 2.7g

Flemish Beef Stew

Points: 6
Serves 4

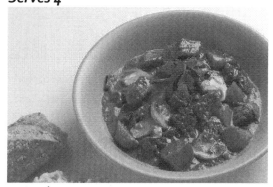

Ingredients
1/2 bay leaf
1/4 teaspoon pepper, freshly ground
Dash teaspoon salt
1/2 teaspoon caraway seeds
3/4 tablespoons Dijon mustard
1/2 clove garlic, minced
1/2 large onion, chopped
2 large carrots or rutabagas, cut into 1-inch pieces
1 cup white wine
1 1/2 tablespoons almond or zucchini flour
6 ounce white button mushrooms, sliced
1 pound bottom round, trimmed of fat and cubed
2 teaspoons canola oil, divided

Directions
1. In a skillet, heat 2 teaspoons of oil over medium heat. Then add beef and brown on all sides for 5 minutes, while turning occasionally.
2. Transfer the meat into a Crockpot, and drain all fat from the pan.
3. Then add 2 teaspoons of oil and brown the rest of the beef. Move it into the Crockpot too.
4. Return the skillet to heat, add mushrooms and cook over medium heat for about 5-7 minutes, while stirring. Remove from heat after the mushrooms gives off their liquid.
5. At this point, sprinkle flour over the cooked mushrooms and cook for 10 seconds, undisturbed. Stir and cook for another 30 seconds.
6. Pour the beer or ale, bring it to a boil as you whisk constantly. Cook for about 3 minutes or until its thickened and bubbling.
7. Pour the mushroom mixture to the Crockpot. Add in caraway seeds, mustard, garlic, onion, carrots, salt, bay leaf and pepper. Stir the ingredients to mix.
8. Lock the lid in place and cook on low heat for around 8 hours. Once ready, open the lid, discard the bay leaf then serve.

Nutritional Information per Serving: 301 Calories; 17g Carbs, 10g Fat, 31g Protein

Slow Cooked Beef & Red Wine Stew

Points: 4

Serves: 4

Ingredients

½ fresh flat-leaf parsley, chopped

1/2 tablespoon butter, unsalted

1/2 cup dry red wine

2 tablespoons tomato paste

Black pepper, freshly ground

Kosher salt

1 1/2 lb. pot roast, trimmed and cut into 4 pieces

1/2 tablespoon canola oil

3 sprigs thyme

2 cloves garlic, chopped

1 large celery rib, chopped

1/2 chopped large red onion

1/2 (8-ounce) package of cremini mushrooms

1/2 lb. carrots or rutabaga cut into small pieces

1/2 teaspoon Dijon mustard

1 ½ tablespoon coconut or almond flour

1 cup beef stock

Directions

1. In a Crockpot, whisk together mustard, flour and beef stock. Add in thyme, garlic, celery, onion, mushrooms and carrots.

2. In a large skillet, heat oil over medium heat then season the beef with pepper and salt.

3. Cook for 10-12 minutes or until browned, while turning occasionally.

4. Transfer the ingredients to a Crockpot. To the skillet, add in tomato paste and cook for a minute, stirring.

5. Add wine and cook for 30 seconds while scrapping up the browned bits. Transfer to a Crockpot.

6. Discard the thyme. Take out the beef and use two forks to shred it. Return to the Crockpot and stir in butter.

7. Cover and cook for 5-6 hours on high or 7 to 8 hours on low. Once tender, serve while topped with parsley.

Nutritional Information per Serving: Calories 477, Protein 39g, Fat 27g, Carbs 14g

Chicken Tikka Masala

Points: 6
Serves 2-3

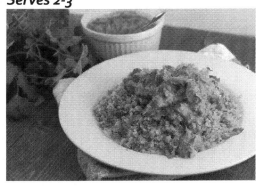

Ingredients
½ fresh cilantro, chopped
1/2 cup coconut milk
1/2 cup heavy cream
5 ounce can tomatoes, diced
2 teaspoons kosher salt
1 teaspoon smoked paprika
2 1/2 teaspoons garam masala
1 1/2 tablespoons tomato paste
1/2 inch ginger root, grated
1 1/2 cloves garlic, minced
1 teaspoon onion powder
1 tablespoon olive oil
1/2 lb. chicken thighs, skinless and boneless
3/4 lbs. (12 ounces) chicken thighs, bone-in skin-on
1/2 teaspoon guar gum

Directions
1. Remove the bones from the chicken thighs and then chop it into bite sized pieces. Do not remove the chicken skin.
2. Add the chicken thigh to a Crockpot or slow cooker and then grate 1 inch of ginger on top.
3. Then add in the tomato paste and canned diced tomatoes into the cooker and combine well.
4. Add in ½ cup of coconut milk and stir well; then cook on high for 3 hours or low for 6 hours.
5. Once done, add guar gum, heavy cream and the coconut cream that remains and mix these into the chicken.
6. Serve topped with preferred veggies or cauliflower rice.
Nutritional Information per Serving: Calories 493, Fats 41.2g, Carbs 7.6g, Protein 26g

Freestyle Soups & Stews

Soups, stews, and the Crock Pot go together like peas and carrots. Throw the ingredients into the pot, set the temperature, and leave it to work wonders! Return from work or leisure to find a delicious, hot soup or stew to enjoy.

Chicken, chili, and lime soupy-stew

Points: 6

Serves: 6

Time: approximately 6 hours

Ingredients:

- 6 chicken thighs, skin on, boneless
- 3 garlic cloves, crushed
- 1 small onion, finely chopped
- 2 tins chopped tomatoes
- 1 red chili, finely chopped
- 1 chicken stock cube
- 2 limes
- Large handful of fresh coriander, chopped

Method:

1. Drizzle some olive oil into the Crock Pot.
2. Place the chicken, garlic, onion, tomatoes, chili, stock cube, juice of 2 limes, 1 cup water, and half the chopped coriander to the pot.
3. Sprinkle with salt and pepper.
4. Place the lid onto the pot and set the temperature to LOW.
5. Cook for 6 hours.
6. Once the soupy-stew has cooked, gently separate the chicken pieces with two forks to shred.
7. Serve while hot, with a couple of slices of avocado on top.

Creamy smoked salmon soup

Points: 5

Serves: 6

Time: approximately 3 hours

Ingredients:

- ½ lb smoked salmon, roughly chopped
- 4 garlic cloves, crushed
- 1 small onion, finely chopped
- 1 leek, finely chopped
- 2 cups heavy cream
- 1 fish stock cube

Method:

1. Drizzle some oil into the Crock Pot.

2. Add the onion, garlic, salmon, leek, stock cube, and 1 cup of water into the pot.
3. Place the lid onto the pot and set the temperature to LOW.
4. Cook for 2 hours.
5. Stir the cream through the soup and continue to cook for a further 1 hour.
6. Serve with a sprinkling of freshly cracked pepper, I don't add extra salt because the smoked salmon is salty enough for me.

Roasted sweet pepper soup

Points: 7
Serves: 6
Time: approximately 4 hours
Ingredients:

- 6 red capsicums, core and seeds removed, roughly chopped
- 2 celery sticks, chopped into chunks
- 6 garlic cloves, finely chopped
- 1 onion, finely chopped
- 1 chicken stock cube
- 1 tsp cumin
- 1 tsp ground coriander
- ½ cup sour cream

Method:

1. Drizzle some olive oil into the Crock Pot.
2. Add the capsicum, celery, garlic, onion, stock cube, cumin, coriander, salt, pepper, and 2 cups of water to the pot.
3. Place the lid onto the pot and set the temperature to LOW.
4. Cook for 6 hours.
5. With a hand-held stick blender, blend the soup until smooth.
6. Stir the sour cream through the soup before serving.
7. Serve while hot.

Lamb and rosemary stew

Points: 4
Serves: 6
Time: approximately 8 hours
Ingredients:

- 2 lb boneless lamb, cut into cubes
- 1 onion, roughly chopped
- 4 garlic cloves, finely chopped
- 2 tsp dried rosemary
- 1 lamb stock cube

Method:

1. Drizzle some olive oil into the Crock Pot.
2. Brown the lamb in an oiled fry pan or skillet for about 2 minutes.

3. Add the lamb, onion, garlic, rosemary, stock cube, salt, pepper, and 3 cups of water to the pot.
4. Place the lid onto the pot and set the time to LOW.
5. Cook for 8 hours.
6. Remove the lid, stir, and serve while hot.

Delicious Beef and onion stew

Points: 5
Serves: 6
Time: approximately 10 hours
Ingredients:

- 2 lb boneless stewing beef, cut into cubes
- 2 onions, roughly chopped
- 5 garlic cloves, crushed
- 1 beef stock cube
- 1 tsp dried mixed herbs

Method:

1. Drizzle the Crock Pot with olive oil.
2. Brown the beef in an oiled fry pan or skillet for about 2 minutes to seal.
3. Place the beef, onions, garlic, stock cube, salt, pepper, herbs, and 3 cups of water to the pot.
4. Place the lid onto the pot.
5. Set the temperature to LOW.
6. Cook for 10 hours.
7. Remove the lid, stir the stew, and serve while hot, with a side of greens and mashed cauliflower.

Freestyle Stewed pork

Points: 7
Serves: 6
Time: approximately 8 hours
Ingredients:

- 2 lb pork loin, cut into cubes
- 1 onion, finely chopped
- 4 garlic cloves, crushed
- 3 cups chicken stock
- 1 tsp dried spices – cumin, coriander, chili, turmeric

Method:

1. Drizzle some olive oil into the Crock Pot.
2. Add the pork, onion, garlic, stock, spices, salt, and pepper to the pot and stir to combine.
3. Place the lid onto the pot and set the temperature to LOW.

4. Cook for 8 hours.
5. Remove the lid, stir, and slightly break the pork apart with 2 forks for a smaller texture.
6. Serve hot with your favorite low-carb veggies!

Coconut, white fish, and fresh coriander soup

Points: 5
Serves: 6
Time: approximately 3 hours
Ingredients:

- 2 lb white fish, cut into chunks
- 4 garlic cloves, crushed
- 1 onion, finely chopped
- 2 tsp fresh ginger, finely grated
- 2 tbsp curry paste (green or red, choose a high-quality paste)
- 3 cups full-fat coconut milk
- 1 lime
- Large handful of fresh coriander, roughly chopped

Method:

1. Drizzle some olive oil into the Crock Pot.
2. Add the fish, garlic, onion, ginger, curry paste, coconut milk, juice of one lime, and half of the coriander to the pot, stir to combine.
3. Place the lid on the pot and set the temperature to LOW.
4. Cook for 5 hours.
5. Remove the lid, stir, and dish into bowls.
6. Sprinkle with the remaining fresh coriander!

Bacon, paprika, and cauliflower soup

Points: 7
Serves: 6
Time: approximately 4 hours
Ingredients:

- 1 large head of cauliflower, cut into chunks
- 4 garlic cloves, crushed
- 1 onion, finely chopped
- 5 slices streaky bacon, cut into small pieces
- 2 cups chicken stock
- 1 tsp smoked paprika
- 1 tsp chili powder (optional)
- 1 cup heavy cream

Method:

1. Drizzle some olive oil into the pot.

2. Add the cauliflower, garlic, onion, bacon, stock, paprika, chili, salt, and pepper to the pot, stir to combine.
3. Place the lid onto the pot and set the temperature to HIGH.
4. Cook for 4 hours.
5. With a hand-held stick blender, blend until smooth.
6. Mix the cream into the soup.
7. Serve while hot, with a sprinkling of paprika on top!

Cheesy broccoli and leek soup

Points: 3
Serves: 6
Time: approximately 3 hours
Ingredients:

- 1 large head of broccoli, cut into small pieces
- 1 large leek, sliced
- 4 garlic cloves, finely chopped
- 2 cups vegetable or chicken stock
- 1 cup grated cheddar cheese
- 1 cup full-fat cream

Method:

1. Drizzle some olive oil into the Crock Pot.
2. Add the broccoli, leek, garlic, stock, salt, and pepper to the pot, stir to combine.
3. Place the lid onto the pot and set the temperature to HIGH.
4. Cook for 3 hours.
5. With a hand-held stick blender, blend the soup until smooth.
6. Add the cheese and cream to the soup and stir.
7. Place the lid back onto the pot and cook on HIGH for another hour, or until the cheese has melted.
8. Serve while hot!

Pumpkin and parmesan soup

Points: 5
Serves: 6
Time: approximately 4 hours
Ingredients:

- 1 butternut pumpkin, peeled and cubed
- 1 onion, finely chopped
- 4 garlic cloves, finely chopped
- 2 cups chicken stock
- ¾ cup grated parmesan cheese
- ½ cup heavy cream

Method:

1. Drizzle some olive oil into the Crock Pot.

2. Add the pumpkin, onion, garlic, stock, salt, and pepper to the pot, stir to combine.
3. Place the lid onto the pot and set the temperature to HIGH.
4. Cook for 4 hours.
5. With a hand-held stick blender, blend until smooth.
6. Stir the parmesan and cream into the hot soup and leave in the pot with the lid on for about twenty minutes, or until the cheese melts.
7. Serve while hot, with an extra grating of parmesan on top!

Chicken and egg soup

Points: 4
Serves: 6
Time: approximately 4 hours
Ingredients:

- 4 chicken thighs, boneless, skinless, cut into medium-sized pieces
- 4 garlic cloves, finely chopped
- 1 red chili, finely chopped
- 1 tbsp finely grated fresh ginger
- 1 lemon
- 4 cups chicken stock
- 6 eggs (1 egg per person)
- Fresh coriander

Method:

1. Drizzle some olive oil into the Crock Pot.
2. Add the chicken, garlic, chili, ginger, juice of one lemon, stock, salt, and pepper to the pot, stir to combine.
3. Place the lid onto the pot and set the temperature to HIGH.
4. Cook for 4 hours.
5. Remove the lid and stir the soup.
6. At this stage, you can either crack the eggs straight into the hot soup to lightly poach, or you can simply poach them in water in a separate pot and place them into each serving bowl of soup.
7. Sprinkle each bowl of soup with fresh coriander!

Beef mince, tomato, and sausage chili

Points: 7, Serves: **6 – 8** , Time: **approximately 8 hours**
Ingredients:

- 2 lb minced beef
- 1 onion, finely chopped
- 4 garlic cloves, crushed
- 4 tomatoes, chopped
- 1 beef stock cube
- 1 tsp smoked paprika
- 1 tsp dried chili flakes (optional)

- 3 sausages, cut into pieces

Method:
1. Drizzle some olive oil into the Crock Pot.
2. Add the minced beef, onion, garlic, tinned tomatoes, stock cube, paprika, chili, sausages, salt, pepper, and one cup of water to the pot, stir to combine.
3. Place the lid onto the pot and set the temperature to LOW.
4. Cook for 8 hours.
5. Remove the lid, stir the chili, and serve while hot!

Chicken and spinach stew

Points: 6, Serves: **6 – 8,** Time: **approximately 8 hours**
Ingredients:
- 2 lb chicken thighs and legs, bone in, skin on
- 2 cups spinach, roughly chopped
- 1 onion, finely chopped
- 6 garlic cloves, crushed
- 1 tsp dried tarragon
- 2 cups chicken stock
- ½ cup dry white wine
- ½ cup heavy cream

Method:
1. Drizzle some olive oil into the Crock Pot.
2. Add the chicken, spinach, onion, 4 cloves of garlic, stock, tarragon, salt, and pepper to the pot, stir to combine.
3. Add the lid to the pot and set the temperature to LOW.
4. Cook for 8 hours.
5. Drizzle some olive oil into a small pot and add the remaining 2 cloves of garlic.
6. Pour the wine into the pot and simmer until reduced.
7. Add the cream to the pot with the wine and stir to combine.
8. Remove the lid from the Crock Pot and stir the wine and cream mixture into the stew.
9. Serve while hot!

Layered "cheeseburger" stew

Points: 7, Serves: **6,** Time: **approximately 4 hours**
Ingredients:
- 2 lb minced beef
- 1 onion, finely chopped
- 4 garlic cloves, crushed
- 1 beef stock cube
- 2 tomatoes, chopped
- ¼ cup sliced pickles or gherkins
- 2 cups grated cheddar cheese
- ½ head of iceberg lettuce, chopped

- 1 fresh tomato, sliced
- Mayonnaise – a dollop on the side of each serving
- Mustard – a dollop on the side of each serving

Method:

1. Drizzle some olive oil into the Crock Pot.
2. Add the minced beef, onion, garlic, stock cube, tinned tomatoes, salt, pepper, and 1 cup of water and stir to combine.
3. Place the lid onto the pot and set the temperature to HIGH.
4. Cook for 4 hours.
5. Remove the lid and stir, place a layer of pickles on top of the beef mince mixture.
6. Sprinkle the cheese over the pickle layer.
7. Place the lid back onto the pot and cook on HIGH for a further 30 minutes, or until the cheese has melted.
8. Serve with a side of shredded iceberg lettuce, freshly sliced tomato, and a dollop of mayonnaise and mustard.

Mozzarella, lamb, and eggplant stew

Points: 5, Serves: **6,** Time: **approximately 8 hours**

Ingredients:

- 2 lb minced lamb
- 1 onion, finely chopped
- 4 garlic cloves, crushed
- 1 large eggplant, cut into small cubes
- 2 tomatoes, chopped
- 1 lamb stock cube
- 1 tsp dried rosemary
- 1 cup grated mozzarella

Method:

1. Drizzle some olive oil into the Crock Pot.
2. Add the minced lamb, onion, garlic, eggplant, stock cube, chopped tomatoes, rosemary, salt and pepper to the pot, stir to combine.
3. Place the lid onto the pot and set the temperature to HIGH.
4. Cook for 8 hours.
5. Remove the lid from the pot and stir the stew.
6. Sprinkle the mozzarella on top of the stew and place the lid back on the pot, cook for a further 30 minutes or until the cheese has melted.
7. Serve hot!

Kale and chicken broth soup

*Points: 6, Serves: 4 – 6, Time: **approximately 4 hours***
Ingredients:

- 6 garlic cloves, finely chopped
- 3 tbsp grated fresh ginger
- 6 cups chicken stock
- 1 large chicken breast, cut into small strips
- 2 cups chopped fresh kale (stalks removed)

Method:

1. Drizzle some olive oil into the Crock Pot.
2. Add the garlic, ginger, stock, chicken breast, kale, salt, and pepper to the pot, stir to combine.
3. Place the lid onto the pot and set the temperature to HIGH.
4. Cook for 4 hours.
5. Serve this soup while steaming hot!.

Freestyle Side Dishes

Cheesy Bacon Cauliflower

Points: 3, Calories: 278 Carbs: 2g Fat: 17g Protein: 6g, Servings: 6, Cooking: 3-4 hour
Ingredients:

3 ounces bacon crumbles
1 ½ C. /350ml grated mozzarella cheese
2 C./500ml milk
¼ tsp./1.25ml pepper
½ tsp./2.5ml salt
¼ C./60ml all-purpose flour
¼ C./60ml butter
2 pounds cauliflower florets
Preparation:

1. Place cauliflower florets into the crockpot.
2. In a pan, melt butter and mix in pepper, salt, and flour. Add milk and simmer until mixture begins to bubble. Add cheese and stir until smooth. Pour over cauliflower and combine.
3. Set to cook on low for 3-4 hours.
4. Mix in bacon. Season as desired.

Crockpot Freestyle Green Beans

Points: 5, Calories: 101 Carbs: 1g Fat: 11g Protein: 4g, Servings: 6, Cooking: 4-5 hours
Ingredients"

14.4-ounce can chicken broth
2 pounds fresh green beans
1 tbsp./15ml butter

2 minced garlic cloves

1 diced yellow onion

Preparation:

1. Sauté garlic and onion together 7-10 minutes. Add to crockpot.
2. Add green beans and chicken broth to crockpot.
3. Set to cook on low for 4-5 hours.
4. Season as needed. Enjoy!

Great Freestyle Stuffing

Points: 5, Calories: 256 Carbs: 2g Fat: 21g Protein: 9g, Servings: 10, Cooking: 3-4 hours

Ingredients:

2 eggs

3-4 C./1l chicken broth

Fresh herbs of choice

¼ C./60ml parsley

12 C. cubed tempeh

2 C./500ml chopped celery

2 diced onions

2 tsp./10ml poultry seasoning

½ tsp./2.5ml salt

½ tsp./2.5ml pepper

1 C./250 ml butter

Preparation:

1. Heat butter in a pan and add pepper, salt, and poultry seasoning. Stir well. Add onions and celery to pan, sautéing till soft. Allow to cool completely.
2. In a bowl, add tempeh cubes with cooled celery and onions. Mix in parsley and chicken broth. Then add in eggs.
3. Cover and chill overnight for tempeh to marinate.
4. Grease your crockpot well. Add stuffing mixture to the pot.
5. Set to cook on low for 3-4 hours.

Pepper Jack Cauliflower

Points: 2, Calories: 272 Carbs: 6g Fat: 21g Protein: 11g, Servings: 6, Cooking: 1 hour

Ingredients:

6 slices cooked and crumbled bacon

4 ounces shredded pepper jack cheese

½ tsp./2.5ml pepper

1 tsp./5ml salt

2 tbsp./30ml butter

¼ C. /60ml whipping cream

4 ounces cream cheese

1 head cauliflower, sliced into 1-inch florets

Preparation:

1. Grease your crockpot.
2. Add all ingredients except pepper jack cheese to crockpot. Stir well.
3. Set to cook on low for 3 hours.
4. Stir in pepper jack cheese and cook another 30-60 minutes until cauliflower is nice and tender.
5. Stir in bacon crumbles and devour!

Parmesan and Chive Mashed Cauliflower

Points: 2, Calories: 190 Carbs: 2g Fat: 18g Protein: 7g, Servings: 4-6, Cooking: 2-3 hours
Ingredients:
¼ C./60ml chopped chives
¼ C./60ml grated parmesan cheese
2 C./500ml chicken broth
2 small cauliflower heads, cored and sliced into florets
Preparation:
1. Add all ingredients to crockpot, stir well.
2. Set to cook on high for 2-3 hours.
3. Season with pepper and salt and sprinkle with additional parmesan.

Celery Root and Cauliflower Puree

Points: 2, Calories: 167 Carbs: 1g Fat: 8g Protein: 4g
Servings: 6-8
Cooking: 5 hours
Ingredients:
3 tbsp./45ml butter
½ tsp./2.5ml salt
1 head cauliflower sliced into florets
1 celery root sliced into ½-inch cubes
Preparation:
1. Add all ingredients to crockpot and combine.
2. Set to cook on high for 5 hours till cauliflower and celery root is tender.
3. With an immersion blender, slightly blend mixture until smooth.

Coconut Lime Cauliflower Rice

Points: 4, Calories: 215 Carbs: 2g Fat: 14g Protein: 8g, Servings: 9, Cooking: 4-5 hours
Ingredients:
2 tsp./10ml lime zest
1 tbsp./15ml chopped cilantro
2 tbsp./30ml water
2 tbsp./30ml coconut oil
3 tbsp./45ml coconut milk powder
2 C./500ml chopped cauliflower
Preparation:
1. Combine all ingredients in your crockpot.

2. Set to cook on high for 4-5 hours.

Delicious Cauliflower Hummus

Calories: 97 Carbs: 0g Fat: 12g Protein: 5g, Servings: 10, Cooking: 4 hours

Ingredients:

¾ tsp./.75ml salt

3 tbsp./45ml extra-virgin olive oil

2 crushed garlic cloves

3 tbsp./45ml lemon juice

1 ½ tbsp./25ml tahini paste

3 garlic cloves

½ tsp./2.5ml salt

2 tbsp./30ml avocado oil

2 tbsp./30ml water

3 C. /750ml cauliflower florets

Preparation:

1. Add all ingredients to your crockpot.
2. Set to cook on high for 4 hours.
3. With an immersion blender, blend mixture until creamy and smooth.

Bacon and Gouda Cauliflower Mash

Points: 3, Calories: 147 Carbs: 2g Fat: 10g Protein: 7g, Servings: 4-6, Cooking: 4 hour

Ingredients:

1/3 C./75 ml shredded smoked gouda cheese

4 slices cooked bacon

¼ tsp./1.25ml garlic powder

¼ tsp./1.25ml pepper

½ tsp./2.5ml salt

2 tbsp./30ml butter

3 tbsp./45ml. heavy cream

4 C./1l cauliflower florets

Preparation:

1. Add all ingredients to your crockpot, combining well.
2. Set to cook on high for 4 hours.
3. With a potato masher, gently mash mixture till just slightly chunky.

Parmesan Zucchini Tots

Points: 5, Calories: 175 Carbs: 1g Fat: 19g Protein: 11g, Servings: 10, Cooking: 3-4 hours

Ingredients:

1 egg

½ C./125ml shredded parmesan cheese

½ tbsp./7.5ml Italian seasoning

1 C./250 ml panko breadcrumbs

1 ½ C./350ml shredded zucchini

Preparation:

1. Add shredded zucchini to crockpot.
2. Combine with remaining ingredients, mixing thoroughly.
3. Set to cook on high for 3-4 hours till zucchini is tender.
4. Remove mixture and shape into small "tot" shapes.
5. Line a sheet with parchment paper and bake 15-20 minutes at 400 degrees till crispy.

Freestyle Appetizers
Curry Spiced Nuts

Points: 2

Serves: 4

Ingredients

Dash cayenne

Kosher salt

Garlic powder

1/2 teaspoon honey

1 3/4 teaspoon coconut oil, melted

1 teaspoon curry powder

1.2 Oz. raw pecan halves

1.2 Oz. raw almonds

1.2 Oz. raw cashews

Directions

1. Mix together all the ingredients in a 6 quart crockpot and stir to incorporate. Cover and cook on high until golden and crisp stirring occasionally. This should take about 1½ to 2 hours.

2. Move the mixture on a parchment paper-lined baking sheet and let cool and dry.

3. Once done, move to an airtight container and keep until ready to serve.

Nutritional Information per Serving: 180 Calories, Proteins 4g, Carbs 6g, Fat 16g

Chuck Roast Stew With Cabbage & Bacon

Points: 3
Serves: 4

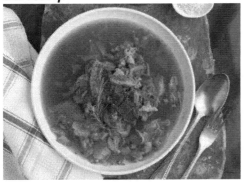

Ingredients

1 /2 cup of homemade beef bone broth

1/2 sprig fresh organic thyme

Fresh ground black pepper to taste

Celtic sea salt

1/2 small organic green or Savoy cabbage

1/2 clove organic garlic, smashed

1 large organic red onion, sliced

1 -1 ½ pound grass-fed chuck roast, cut in 2" pieces

1/4 pound of organic uncured bacon, in strips

Directions

1. Add the ingredients to the crockpot beginning with bacon slices, onion slices and garlic in the bottom.

2. Follow with chuck roast, cabbage slices, thyme and homemade broth.

3. Now season with Celtic salt and a sufficient amount of ground pepper.

4. Cook the mixture for 7 hours or low heat setting. Then serve in bowls and enjoy.

Nutritional Information per Serving: Calories 408.4, Fat 24.5g, Carbs 4.9g, Protein 39.6g

Slow Cooker Garlicky Shrimp

Points: 2

Serves: 3

Ingredients

1/2 tablespoon flat-leaf parsley, minced

1 pound extra-large raw shrimp, peeled and deveined

1/8 teaspoon crushed red pepper flakes

1/8 teaspoon black pepper, freshly ground

1/2 teaspoon kosher salt

1/2 teaspoon smoked Spanish paprika

3 cloves garlic, thinly sliced

6 tablespoons extra-virgin olive oil

Directions

1. Mix together crushed pepper flakes, black pepper, salt, paprika, garlic and oil in a crockpot. Stir the mixture to incorporate.

2. Then cover and cook for 30 minutes on high heat settings. Now stir in shrimp to coat it then cover and cook for another 10 minutes.

3. Stir to help the shrimp cook evenly until all of the fish meat is opaque or for about 10 minutes or so.

4. Move the fish and its sauce to a serving dish then sprinkle with parsley to garnish. Serve it warm.

Nutritional Information per Serving: Calories 210, Fat 12g, Carbs 2g, Protein 23g

Cantaloupe and Cucumber Salad

Points: 4
Serves: 4

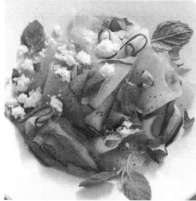

Ingredients

1 tablespoon snipped fresh mint
1 tablespoon snipped fresh basil
3 tablespoons crumbled feta cheese
1/2 large cucumber, halved lengthwise and sliced
1/2 large cantaloupe, cubed
For Balsamic Vinaigrette
1 tablespoon olive oil
1/4 teaspoon black pepper
1/4 teaspoon salt
1 tablespoon white balsamic vinegar
Directions

1. First prepare the balsamic vinaigrette by whisking together black pepper, salt and balsamic vinegar.

2. Then whisk in olive oils and mix together. This makes about 2 tablespoons of dressing.

3. Toss together mint, basil, feta cheese, cucumber and cantaloupe in a large bowl.

4. Then drizzle the dressing over the mixture and toss. Serve and enjoy.

Nutritional Information per Serving: Calories 79, Carbs 7g, Fat 5g, Proteins 2g

Blueberry Lemon Custard Cake

Points: 6, Calories: 375 Carbs: 4g Fat: 27g Protein: 14g, Servings: 8-9, Cooking: 3 hours

Ingredients:

½ C./125ml fresh blueberries

2 C./500ml light cream

½ tsp./2.5ml salt

½ C. /125ml sweetener of choice

1 tsp./5ml lemon stevia

1/3 C./75 ml lemon juice

2 tsp./10ml lemon zest

½ C./125ml coconut flour

6 separated eggs

Preparation:

1. Into a stand mixer, add egg whites. Whip till soft peaks are created. Set to the side.
2. Whisk yolks with remaining ingredients minus blueberries. Fold in egg whites.
3. Grease crockpot and pour in batter. Sprinkle with blueberries.
4. Set to cook on low for 3 hours.
5. Allow to cook at least 1 hour and then chill at least 2 hours or overnight.
6. Serve ice cold with sugar-free whipped cream!

Freestyle Chocolate Cake

Points: 7, Calories: 357 Carbs: 5g Fat: 26g Protein: 13g, Servings: 6-7, Cooking: 2 ½ hours

Ingredients:

1/3 C./75ml sugar-free chocolate chips

¾ tsp./1.75ml vanilla extract

2/3 C./150ml unsweetened almond milk

6 tbsp./90ml melted butter

3 eggs

¼ tsp./1.25ml salt

1 ½ tsp./25ml baking powder

3 tbsp./45ml whey protein powder

½ C. /125ml cocoa powder

½ C./125ml Swerve

1 C./250 ml + 2 tbsp. almond flour

Preparation:

1. Grease crockpot.
2. Mix salt, baking powder, protein powder, cocoa powder, sweetener, and almond flour together.
3. Mix in vanilla, almond milk, eggs, and butter. Fold in chocolate chips.
4. Pour into crockpot.
5. Set to cook on low for 2 ½ hours.
6. Let cool and then slice into pieces.

Whole 30 Crock-Pot Beef Stew

Points: 6
Serves 4

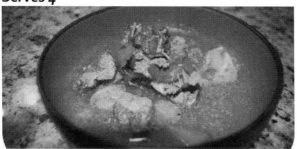

Ingredients
Cilantro
4 cups chicken broth
29 oz. can of peeled tomatoes, crushed
2 tomatoes, quartered
1/2 teaspoon cayenne pepper
1 teaspoon parsley
1½ teaspoons oregano
3 garlic cloves
3 lbs. beef stew meat
4 medium rutabagas
5 radishes
3 celery sticks
1 onion

Directions
1. Start by placing the quartered rutabagas, carrots, celery and chopped onions in a Crockpot or slow cooker,
2. Then add in the meat and cover with chicken broth, tomatoes and spices.
3. Cook the mixture on low for 8 hours or high for 4 hours. You can use cilantro for garnish.

Nutritional Information per Serving: Calories 324.9, Fat 9.7g, Carbs 18.6g, Protein 40.5g

Philly Cheese Steaks

Points: 7
Serves 3

Ingredients
1 1/2 slices low-fat provolone cheese
Freestyle zucchini bread
10 tablespoons low sodium beef broth
1/4 tablespoon marinara sauce
1/2 green bell pepper, sliced
2 ounces button mushrooms, sliced
1/4 teaspoon kosher salt

1/8 teaspoon pepper

1/4 tablespoon butter

6 ounce lean sirloin steak, sliced

1/4 tablespoon olive oil

1/4 garlic clove, minced

1/2 green onions, sliced

Directions

1. Start by placing the olive oil, garlic and onions in a crockpot then stir to coat the vegetables in oil.

2. Add in butter and the steak, and season with salt and pepper.

3. Now add in bell peppers and mushrooms, along with broth and marinara sauce.

4. Cover the crockpot and cook for 5-6 hours on high and 6-8 hours on low.

5. To make the sandwich, simply add the cheese-steak mixture to a friendly bread, and top with the provolone cheese.

6. Lightly toast to melt the cheese, and then serve.

Nutritional Information per Serving: Calories 314, Carbs 22g, Fat 16g, Protein: 20g

Sugar-Free Pumpkin Pie Bars

Points: 6

Servings 4

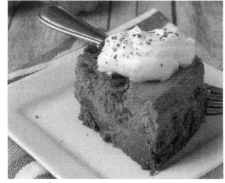

Ingredients

Crust

1 tablespoon butter softened

1 tablespoon Swerve

Dash teaspoon salt

2 tablespoons sunflower seed flour

1 tablespoon cocoa powder, unsweetened

3 tablespoons shredded coconut, unsweetened

Filling

1 teaspoon pure stevia extract

1 teaspoon cinnamon liquid stevia

1 tablespoon pumpkin pie spice

1 tablespoon vanilla extract

1/2 teaspoon salt

6 eggs

1 cup heavy cream

1 29 ounce can pumpkin puree

Directions

1. Add all ingredients in a food processor then puree to obtain fine crumbs. Then grease the bottom of a slow cooker.

2. Now press the crust mixture onto the bottom of the slow cooker evenly.

3. Then add the filling ingredients to a mixer and mix until well incorporated.

4. At this point, pour the filling mixture on the crust and cover the crockpot. Cook on low heat for 3 about hours.

5. Once done, uncover the lid and allow to cool for about 30 minutes. Keep it chilled for round 3 hours and then slice to serve.

Nutritional Information per Serving: Calories 151, Fat 12.4g, Carbs 6.2g, Protein 5.4g

Lemon Crock Pot Cake

Points: 5, Calories: 310 Carbs: 4g Fat: 29g Protein: 8g, Servings: 8, Cooking: 2-3 hours

Ingredients:

2 eggs

Zest of 2 lemons

2 tbsp./30ml lemon juice

½ C./125ml whipping cream

½ C./125ml melted butter

½ tsp./2.5ml xanthan gum

2 tsp./10ml baking powder

3 tbsp./45ml swerve sweetener

½ C./125ml coconut flour

1 ½ C./350ml almond flour

Topping:

2 tbsp./30ml lemon juice

2 tbsp./30ml melted butter

½ C./125ml boiling water

3 tbsp./45ml swerve sweetener

Preparation:

1. Combine xanthan gum, baking powder, sweetener, and flours together.
2. Whisk egg, lemon juice and zest, whipping cream, and butter together.
3. Combine wet and dry mixtures together till well incorporated. Pour into a greased crockpot.
4. For topping, combine all topping components till incorporated and spread over top of cake mixture.
5. Set to cook on high for 2-3 hours.
6. Serve warm with whipped cream and fresh fruit!

Chocolate Molten Lava Cake

Points: 7, Calories: 418 Carbs: 4g Fat: 27g Protein: 8g, Servings: 12, Cooking: 3 hours

Ingredients:

2 C./500ml hot water

4 ounces sugar-free chocolate chips

½ tsp./2.5ml vanilla liquid stevia

1 tsp./5ml vanilla extract

3 egg yolks

3 whole eggs

½ C./125ml melted and cooled butter

1 tsp./5ml baking powder

½ tsp./2.5ml salt

5 tbsp./60ml unsweetened cocoa powder

½ C./125ml flour

1 ½ C./350ml swerve sweetener

Preparation:

1. Grease crockpot liberally.
2. Whisk baking powder, salt, 3 tbsp. cocoa powder, flour, and 1 ¼ C. swerve together.
3. Stir liquid stevia, vanilla, yolks, eggs, and melted butter together.
4. Combine wet and dry mixture till well incorporated. Pour into crockpot.
5. Top with chocolate chips. Mix in the remaining swerve and cocoa powder.
6. Set to cook on low for 3 hours.

Freestyle Pumpkin Custard

Points: 4, Calories: 419 Carbs: 4g Fat: 16g Protein: 19g, Servings: 8-10, Cooking: 2-3 hours

Ingredients:

4 tbsp./60ml butter

1/8 tsp./25ml salt

1 tsp./5ml pumpkin pie spice

½ C./125ml almond flour

1 tsp./5ml vanilla extract

1 C./250 ml pumpkin puree

½ C./125ml granulated stevia

4 eggs

Preparation:

1. Grease inside of crockpot.
2. Beat eggs until smooth. Then beat in sweetener gradually. Add vanilla and pumpkin puree until blended well.
3. Then mix in pumpkin pie spice, salt, and almond flour. Blend as you add in butter. Pour into crockpot.
4. Place a paper towel over the opening of the pot before closing it.

5. Set to cook on low 2 – 2 ¾ hours.
6. Serve warm with whipped cream and a dash of nutmeg!

Blackberry Chocolate Chip Cake

Points: 3, Calories: 289 Carbs: 5g Fat: 19g Protein: 9g, Servings: 10-12, Cooking: 3 hours

Ingredients:

1/3 C./75 ml dark chocolate chips (sugar-free)

1 C./250 ml blackberries

½ C./125ml heavy cream

¼ C./60ml melted butter

¼ C./60ml melted coconut oil

4 eggs

¼ tsp./1.25ml salt

2 tsp./10ml baking soda

¼ C./125ml chocolate whey protein powder

½ swerve sweetener

1 C./250 ml unsweetened shredded coconut

2 C./500ml almond flour

Preparation:

1. Grease inside of crockpot with butter.
2. Mix all of the dry ingredients together. Then add in all wet components, blending well to ensure adequate incorporation.
3. Pour batter into prepared crockpot.
4. Set to cook on low for 3 hours.
5. Serve topped with more blackberries!

Crockpot Freestyle Apple Cider

Points: 2, Calories: 178 Carbs: 1g Fat: 8g Protein: 5g, Servings: 12-15, Cooking: 3 hours

Ingredients:

7 C. water

¼ C./60ml maple syrup

¼ C./60ml coconut sugar

1 tsp./5ml allspice berries

2 tsp./10ml whole cloves

3 cinnamon sticks

1 sliced naval orange

6 apples of choice, cored and sliced

Preparation:

1. Pour all ingredients into your crockpot and pour water over everything.
2. Set to cook on high for 3 hours.
3. Discard orange slices and cinnamon sticks.
4. With an immersion blender, blend mixture until smooth.
5. Cook for another hour on high.

6. Strain mixture through cheesecloth.
7. Add back to the pot to keep warm.

Freestyle Zesty Lemon Cake

Points: 6, Calories: 250 Carbs: 2g Fat: 16g Protein: 11g, Servings: 10, Cooking: 6-8 hours

Ingredients:

Zest of 1 lemon

4 eggs

½ C./125ml unsweetened almond milk

1/3 C./75 mlbutter

1 tsp./5ml baking soda

2 tsp./10ml cream of tartar

2 tsp./10ml vanilla extract

½ C./125ml swerve sweetener

¼ C./60ml plain egg protein powder

¼ C./60ml coconut flour

2 C./500ml almond flour

Filling:

1 C./250 ml low-carb lemon curd

1 tsp./5ml vanilla extract

1 C./250 ml coconut cream

Glaze:

2 tbsp./30ml swerve sweetener

Zest of 1 lemon

1 tbsp./15ml lemon juice

2 tbsp./30ml coconut oil

½ C./125ml coconut butter

Preparation:

1. Combine almond milk and butter together. Then mix in vanilla, eggs, and lemon zest.
2. Combine all dry components together. Then combine wet and dry mixtures, combining well.
3. Line a springform pan with parchment paper and pour batter into it.
4. Place pan into the crockpot and cook on low for 2 hours.
5. Take out and place in fridge 4-6 hour to chill.
6. To prepare filling, combine all ingredients together until smooth. Do the same with glaze.
7. Cut cake in half. Fill one part of the cake with filling, lay other half over the top and then drizzle with glaze. Tip with additional lemon zest.

Chicken with Lemon Parsley Butter

Points: 4, Serves: 3

Ingredients

1 tablespoon fresh parsley, chopped

2 tablespoon butter or ghee

1/2 whole lemon, sliced thinly

1/8 teaspoon ground black pepper

1/4 teaspoon kosher salt

1/2 cup water

1/2 whole roasting chicken

Directions

1. Wash and pat dry the meat and discard any innards.

2. Season the chicken with pepper and salt then put it at the center of a slow cooker.

3. Pour some water along with the meat to just cover the bottom of the cooking pot.

4. Cook the chicken for 3 hours on high or longer in case you're cooking a bigger chicken.

5. Serve once the juices are clear and the meat is no longer pink. The internal temperature should reach around 165 degrees F.

6. You may choose to add lemon slices, parsley and butter 10 minutes before serving or instead cook them in a small pan. Cook until the lemon darkens in color and the butter melts then pour over the cooked chicken.

Nutritional Information per Serving: Calories 300, Fat 18g, Carbs 1g, Protein 29g

Crockpot Brownie Bites

Points: 6

Servings 4

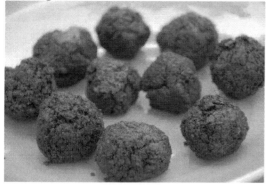

Ingredients

2 tablespoons brewed coffee or water

1 teaspoons pure vanilla extract

1/2 cup coconut oil melted

3 ¼ tablespoons coconut milk, unsweetened

1 egg

1/2 teaspoon salt

1 teaspoons baking soda

1 teaspoons baking powder

4 ¾ tablespoons cocoa powder, unsweetened

6 1/2 tablespoons coconut sugar

12 ¾ tablespoons almond flour, blanched

Directions

1. First use coconut oil to grease the slow cooker.

2. Then mix all ingredients and spread them evenly on the cooker.

3. Cook the mixture for 4-5 hours until well cooked through.

4. At this point, allow to cool for 30 minutes then scoop out using a large spoon or cookie scoop. Make it into balls.

5. Scoop the snack with caramel glaze if you like.

Nutritional Information per Serving: Calories 326.1, Fat 24.1g, Carbs 27.8g, Protein 7.2g

Slow Cooker Turkey Wedges

Points: 7
Serves: 4

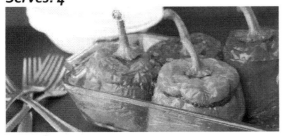

Ingredients

¼ 6 -inches low carb gluten-free bread

1/8 small cucumber, seeded and chopped

1/8 teaspoon black pepper

1 1/3 tablespoon bottled marinara sauce

3.625 ounce diced tomatoes with juices, no-salt-added

3/4 cloves garlic, minced

3 tablespoons finely chopped red onion

1/4 pound lean ground turkey

Nonstick cooking spray

Directions

1. Coat a skillet with cooking spray then cook turkey, garlic and ½ cup onion in the skillet for 5-8 minutes over medium-high heat. Remember to stir occasionally.

2. As soon as the onion is tender and the turkey has browned, stir in tomatoes, pepper and barbecue sauce.

3. Move the mixture to a Crockpot and cover. Keep it warm for 2 hours through the keep-warm settings.

4. Sprinkle the contents of the slow cooker with cucumber and chopped onion then serve the turkey with Pita wedges.

5. To make the wedges, preheat your oven to 350 degrees. Then split pita bread in half, and cut each half into 8 wedges.

6. Arrange the wedges on a baking sheet and bake for 10-15 minutes. Once crisp and lightly browned, allow to cool.

Nutritional Information per Serving: Calories 80, Carbs 8g, Total Fat 2g, Proteins 7g

<u>*Slow Cooker Stuffed Peppers*</u>

Points: 5
Serves 4

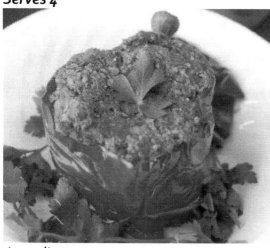

Ingredients

1/4 cup beef stock
Salt and pepper to taste
1/4 cup Italian seasoning blend
6 ounces tomato paste
4 cloves of garlic, minced
1 radish, diced
1 onion, diced
1/2 head of cauliflower
1 lb. ground meat
4 bell peppers

Directions

1. In a food processor, pulse garlic, carrots, onion and cauliflower until fine.

2. Then cut off the top of peppers, and keep them intact. Also clean the seeds out.

3. In a mixing bowl, combine pepper, salt, seasonings, tomato paste, meat and vegetables and then spoon this mixture into the peppers. Try to level the peppers off at the top and position them in the slow cooker.

4. Now place the tops of the peppers on them. Pour the liquid into the bottom of the slow cooker, and then cook the mixture on low for about 6-8 hours.

5. Serve topped with preferred ingredients.

Nutritional Information per Serving: Calories 380.4, Fat 20.6g, Carbs 15.9g, Protein 33.7g

Tasty Caramelized Onions

Points: 6
Serves: 4

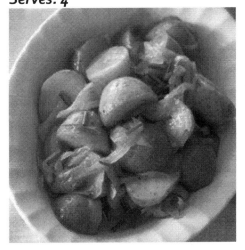

Ingredients
1/8 teaspoon ground black pepper
1/8 teaspoon salt
1 tablespoon packed brown sugar
1/4 cup beef or chicken broth, reduced-sodium
1 tablespoon butter, melted
3/4 pounds rutabagas, halved
1 large green onion
Directions
1. Mix together rutabagas and onions in a slow cooker.
2. Mix together pepper, salt, brown sugar, broth and melted butter in a small bowl. Pour the mixture over the rutabagas and onion mixture.
3. Cook on high heat for 3 to 3 ½ hours or under low heat for 6-7 hours, while stirring at least once.
4. Use a slotted spoon to serve. You cans spoon a little of the cooking juices over the rutabagas to moisten, or sprinkle some more pepper if you like it.
Nutritional Information per Serving: Calories 131, Carbs 25g, Total Fat 3g, Proteins 3g

Homemade Greek Yogurt

Points: 6
Serves: 4

Ingredients

½ cup plain full-fat yogurt
½ gallon whole milk

Directions

1. To make Greek yoghurt, line a fine mesh using 3 layers of cheesecloth, then put it in a large bowl.
2. Move the yoghurt to a sieve and allow the liquid whey to drain so that you can get preferred yoghurt consistency. This should take around 4 hours.
3. Chill the yoghurt and then serve.

Nutritional Information per Serving: Calories 220, Proteins 20g, Carbs 9g, Fat 11g

Freestyle Dessert

Crock Pot Cabbage Rolls

Points: 4, Serves 3 cabbage rolls

Ingredients

1/4 cup of marinara sauce, unsweetened
1/8 teaspoon of pepper
Few sprigs of fresh parsley, chopped
1/4 teaspoon of onion powder
1/2 minced garlic cloves
1/4 cup good quality parmesan cheese
1/4 pound of ground beef
3 large cabbage leaves

Directions

1. First cook the cabbage leaves in a microwave or stovetop for 3 to 5 minutes to soften them.
2. Then put half of the sauce into the crockpot. In a medium bowl, mix together ground beef, minced garlic, parmesan, parsley and pepper.
3. Soon after the cabbage leaves have cooled down, measure about ¼ cup of the meat mixture into the cabbage leaf.
4. Then bring together the sides of the leaf over the meat filling and then roll the leaf up to create a cabbage roll.
5. Put each cabbage roll into a crockpot the seam side facing down. Top the roll with the rest of marinara sauce and then cook on high for about 5 minutes.

Nutritional Information per Serving: Calories 177.5, Fat 13.4 g, Carbs 3.6g, Protein 10.4g

Slow Cooker Cheesecake

Points: 6
Serves 4

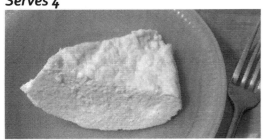

Ingredients
1/4 tablespoon vanilla
1/2 cup Splenda
1 1/2 eggs
1 ½ -8 oz. packages cream cheese

Directions
1. Allow the cream cheese to warm up then put it in a large bowl. Add in a sweetener.
2. Using a mixer, combine cream cheese and the sweetener until well incorporated.
3. Then add in eggs one by one, and mix to blend. Now coat the slow cooker bowl with cooking spray and then pour the cream cheese.
4. Add a few cups of water to the slow cooker to last for 2 hours and then put the cheesecake into the cooking bowl.
5. Close the lid in place and cook on high heat for about 2 to 2 ½ hours.
6. If the mixture puffs up at any time of the cooking, let cooking progress for about 2 hours. Cook until a knife inserted in the mixture comes out clean.

Nutritional Information per Serving: Calories 317.1, Fat 31.0g, Carbs 9.7g Protein 8.4g

Slow Cooker Dark Chocolate Cake

Points: 7
Serves 4

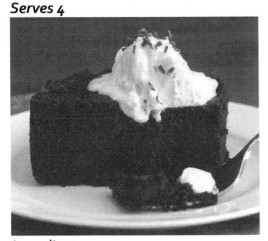

Ingredients
2 tablespoons sugar-free chocolate chips

1/3 teaspoon vanilla extract

4 ¼ tablespoons unsweetened almond milk

2 1/2 tablespoon butter, melted

1 large egg

Dash teaspoon salt

3/5 teaspoon baking powder

1 1/4 tablespoon egg white protein powder, unflavored

3 ¼ tablespoons cocoa powder

3 ¼ tablespoons cocoa powder

3 ¼ tablespoons, Granular

7 1/4 tablespoons almond flour

Directions

1. Grease a crockpot and set aside. Whisk together almond flour, salt, baking powder, protein powder, cocoa powder and the sweetener in a medium bowl.

2. Then stir in eggs, butter, vanilla extract and almond milk until well incorporated. Stir in chocolate if you like to include it.

3. Pour the batter into the crockpot's insert and cook for about 2 -2 ½ hours on low heat.

4. Once you achieve cake consistency, turn off the cooker and allow to cool for about 20 to 30 minutes.

5. Finally cut into pieces and serve it when hot or warm. Serve with unsweetened whipped cream.

Nutritional Information per Serving: Calories 205, Fat 16.97g, Carbs 8.42g Protein 7.37g

Sugar Free Chocolate Molten Lava Cake

Points: 7

Serves 3

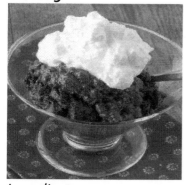

Ingredients

1/2 cup hot water

1 ounce chocolate chips, sugar free

1/4 teaspoon vanilla liquid stevia

1/4 teaspoon vanilla extract

1 egg yolk

1 whole egg

2 tablespoons butter melted, cooled

1/4 teaspoon baking powder

1/8 teaspoon salt

3 ¾ teaspoons cocoa powder, unsweetened

2 tablespoons almond flour

6 tablespoons Swerve sweetener divided

Directions

1. Coat the slow cooker with grease. Then whisk together flour, baking powder, 2 tablespoons cocoa powder, almond flour and 4 tablespoons of Swerve in a bowl.

2. In a separate bowl, stir in eggs with melted butter, liquid stevia, vanilla extract, egg yolks and eggs.

3. Now add the wet ingredients to the dry ones and combine to fully incorporate. Pour the mixture into the slow cooker.

4. Top the mixture with chocolate chips. In a separate bowl, whisk together the remaining swerve with cocoa powder and hot water and pour this mixture over chocolate chips.

5. Cover the slow cooker and cook on low for around 3 hours. Once done, let cool and then serve.

Nutritional Information per Serving: Calories 157, Fat 13g, Carbs 10.5g, Protein 3.9g

Blueberry Lemon Custard Cake

Points: 6

Serves 3

Ingredients

2 tablespoons fresh blueberries

1/2 cup light cream

1/8 teaspoon salt

2 tablespoons Swerve sweetener

1/4 teaspoon lemon liquid stevia

1 1/3 tablespoon lemon juice

1/2 teaspoon lemon zest

2 tablespoons coconut flour

1 ½ eggs separated

Directions

1. Put egg whites into a stand mixture and whip to achieve stiff peaks consistency.

2. Set the egg whites aside then whisk the yolks along with the other ingredients apart from the blueberries.

3. Fold the egg whites into the batter to fully combine, and then grease the slow cooker.

4. Now pour the mixture into the pot and top with the blue berries. Cover the crockpot and cook on low for about 3 hours. When cooked through, a toothpick inserted in the cake should come out clean.

5. Let cool when not covered for 1 hour then keep it chilled for at least 2 hours or overnight.

6. Serve the cake topped with unsweetened cream if you like.

Nutritional Information per Serving: Calories 140, Fat 9.2g, Carbs 7.3g, Protein 3.9g

Slow Cooker Bread Pudding

Points: 5
Serves 4

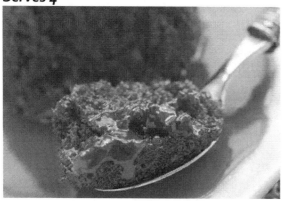

Ingredients
1 tablespoons raisins
1/2 teaspoon cinnamon
1 1/2 teaspoon vanilla extract
1/4 cup swerve
1 egg white
1 whole egg
1 1/2 cups almond milk
4 slices pumpkin bread, recipe included

Directions
1. Cut the bread into pieces. Then mix all the ingredients in the crockpot.
2. Cook the mixture on high heat until the liquid is soaked up by the bread, or for 4 to 5 hours.

Nutritional Information per Serving: Calories 182, Fat 2g, Carbs 11g, Protein 8g

Tiramisu Bread Pudding

Points: 5
Serves 4

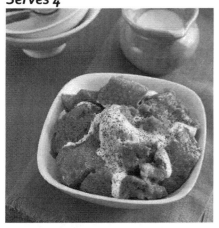

Ingredients
3/4 teaspoons unsweetened cocoa
1/3 teaspoon vanilla extract
2 tablespoons mascarpone cheese
Cooking spray
3 1/4 cups bread
1 large egg, lightly beaten
6.4 ounces of almond milk, divided
3/4 tablespoons Kahlua (coffee-flavored liqueur)
1 3/4 teaspoons instant espresso granules
2 tablespoons coconut sugar
1.6 ounce (47.3ml) water

Directions
1. Mix together water, coconut sugar and instant espresso granules in a small saucepan.
2. Bring to a boil, stirring for about 1 minute until well incorporated, and then remove from heat. Stir in the Kahlua liqueur.
3. In a large bowl, mix together eggs and almond milk and whisk together. Add in the espresso mixture, and whisk to combine.
4. Now pour the friendly bread into a casserole that is coated with oil or cooking spray.
5. Put the dish in a crockpot and cover. Cook the mixture on low for around 2 hours or until well cooked.
6. Mix together vanilla, mascarpone cheese and the remaining almond milk in a bowl then whisk to blend.
7. Finally spoon the bread pudding into your preferred dessert dishes and top with mascarpone sauce if you like. Garnish with cocoa and serve.

Nutritional Information per Serving: Calories 199, Fat 9g, Protein 6.7g, Carbs 9g

Crock Pot Sugar-Free Dairy Free Fudge

Points: 5
Serves 3

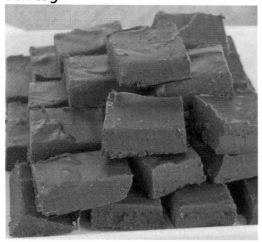

Ingredients
A dash of salt
Dash of pure vanilla extract
½ tablespoon coconut milk
4 tablespoons sugar-free chocolate chips
1/4 teaspoons vanilla liquid stevia
Directions
1. In a slow cooker pot, stir in coconut milk, stevia, vanilla, chocolate chips and salt.
2. Cover the crockpot and cook on low for about 2 hours. Once done cooking, uncover and let sit for about 30 minutes undisturbed.
3. Then stir well for about 5 minutes or until smooth. Using parchment paper, line a casserole dish and then spread the mixture in.
4. Keep refrigerated until firm, or for around 30 minutes or so.
Nutritional Information Per Serving: Calories 65, Fat 5g, Carbs 2g, Protein 1g

Cheesy Cauliflower Garlic Bread

Points: 3
Serves 4
Ingredients
2 tablespoons chopped fresh basil
1 clove garlic, minced
1/4 teaspoon pepper
1/4 teaspoon salt
1½ tablespoons coconut flour
1 cup shredded mozzarella, divided
1 large egg

6 ounces cauliflower florets

Directions

1. Grease a crockpot and set aside. Then chop the cauliflower in a food processor to obtain rice consistency. Move to a large bowl.

2. Then stir in pepper, salt, coconut flour, eggs and a cup of shredded cheese then to stir to blend.

3. Now press the mixture into the bottom of the greased crockpot. Then sprinkle the remaining cheese along with garlic.

4. Once done, cook on high until the edges are crisp and browned and the cheese has melted, or for about 2-4 hours.

5. At this point, cut the bread into slices and remove from the crockpot. Sprinkle with basil and enjoy.

Nutritional Information per Serving: Calories 224, Fat 14.95g, Carbs 5.63g, Protein 15.29g

Healthy Buffalo Chicken Dip

Points: 2
Serves 3

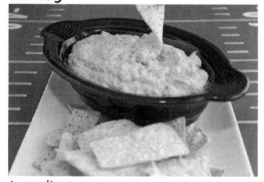

Ingredients

1/4 cup mozzarella cheese

1/2 cups cooked shredded chicken

8 teaspoons frank's red hot sauce

1/2 tablespoon ranch dips seasoning

1/4 cup 0% Greek yogurt

2.5 oz. Neufchatel cream cheese

Directions

1. In a slow cooker, add in all the ingredients preferably lined to make it easier to clean.

2. Cook on low for about 3 to 4 hours, while stirring at regular interval of 1 hour.

3. Serve and enjoy the dessert.

Nutritional Information per Serving: Calories 444.4, Fat 29.1g, Carbs 12.5g, Protein 32.2g

Freestyle Zucchini Bread

Points: 3
Serves 4

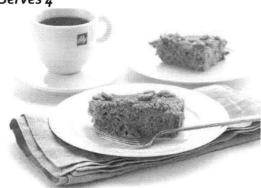

Ingredients

1/2 teaspoon vanilla extract

1/4 cup water

1/4 cup coconut oil

3 large eggs

1/4 teaspoon nutmeg

1/2 teaspoon ginger

2 teaspoon cinnamon

2 teaspoon baking powder

1/4 cup egg white protein powder, unflavored

1/2 cup Swerve Sweetener

2/3 cup shredded coconut

1 1/3 cups almond flour

1/2 teaspoon salt

2 1/2 cups shredded zucchini

Directions

1. Put the zucchini in a sieve over a sink or bowl. Season with salt and allow to drain for about 1 hour.

2. Squeeze out as much fluid as possible and then set aside. Meanwhile, grease your crockpot's insert.

3. Whisk together shredded coconut, almond flour, nutmeg, ginger, cinnamon, baking powder, protein powder and a sweetener in a large bowl.

4. Stir in melted butter, eggs, zucchini, vanilla extract and water until well combined.

5. At this point, spread the mixture in a crockpot, cover and cook for 2 ½ to 3 hours on low heat setting.

6. Then let cool inside the crockpot and then slice and enjoy.

Nutritional Information per Serving: Calories 238, Fat 20.22g, Carbs 6.91g, Protein 8.95g

Buffalo Chicken Dip

Points: 4
Serves 4

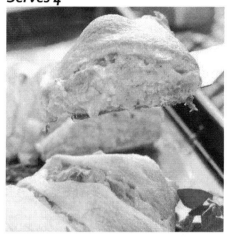

Ingredients
6 tablespoons pepper sauce
3/4 cups shredded Cheddar cheese
1/2 (10-ounce) cans of drained chunk chicken
1 (8-ounce) package cream cheese, softened
1/2 bunch of cleaned celery, chopped
1/2 cup ranch dressing
Directions
1. Over medium heat, start by heating the chicken as well as the hot sauce inside a skillet until they are heated through.
2. Next, star the ranch dressing and cream cheese in then cook while stirring until they are nicely blended and warm.
3. Once done with the previous step, mix ½ of the shredded cheese then proceed to transfer your prepared mixture into a crockpot.
4. You can sprinkle some of the extra cheese on top, cover and set the cook setting to low then cook until it is hot and bubbly.
5. Serve with celery sticks if you like.
Nutritional Information per Serving: Calories 530.0, Fat 42.5g, Carbs 8.1g, Protein 27.4g

Poppy Seed-Lemon Bread

Points:56
Serves 3

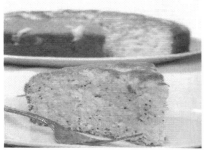

Ingredients

1/2 cups almond flour
1/4 tablespoon baking powder
1 tablespoon poppy seeds
1 egg
1/4 cup coconut sugar
1/8 teaspoon salt
2 tablespoons vegetable oil
3 tablespoons tofu (puree)
1/4 cup almond milk
3/4 cup plain Greek-style yogurt or sour cream
1/4 cup fresh lemon juice
3/4 teaspoon finely shredded lemon peel
1/4 teaspoon vanilla

Directions

1. Begin by coating your Crockpot with non-stick cooking spray.
2. Then combine poppy seeds, flour, salt and baking powder in a large bowl, mix and set aside.
3. In a medium bowl, stir together the tofu puree, sugar, oil, milk, yogurt, lemon juice, lemon peel and vanilla until blended.
4. Now add the sugar mixture to the flour mix, and stir until lightly lumpy.
5. Spoon the batter into your Crockpot. Cover and cook on high for 1 ½ to 2 hours, or until set.
6. Once done, turn off the heat, and remove the lid. Cover the opening with paper towels and place the lid on top.
7. Leave for 10-15 minutes to cool.
8. To serve, simply run a knife over the edges of the slow cooker. Then take out the bread from the cooker, and cool completely on a wire rack.
9. Serve and enjoy.

Nutritional Information per Serving: Calories 295.6, Fat 24.3g, Carbs 17.9g, Protein 6.0g

Nutmeg-Infused Pumpkin Bread

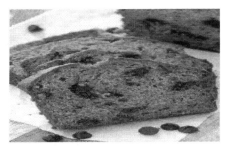

Points: 6

Serves 4

Ingredients

0.5 oz. unsalted pecan pieces, toasted
1/4 tablespoon pure vanilla extract
1 tablespoon safflower oil
1 egg white
2 tablespoons plain Greek yogurt
1/4 cup cooked and puréed pumpkin
1/8 teaspoon sea salt
Dash ground allspice
1/4 teaspoon ground nutmeg
Dash teaspoon baking soda
1/2 teaspoon baking powder
2 tablespoons coconut sugar
7 tablespoons almond flour
2 tablespoons dried apple cranberries, unsweetened
3 tablespoons 100% apple juice, plain
Olive oil cooking spray

Directions

1. Lightly grease a non-stick loaf pan with cooking spray. Set aside.
2. Mix together cranberries and apple juice in a small saucepan. Heat the mixture on high to boil, then remove from heat and let cool for around 10 minutes.
3. Then mix together nutmeg, baking soda, allspice, baking powder, salt, maple sugar flakes and flour in a large bowl. Set aside.
4. Now mix vanilla, oil, egg whites, yoghurt, pumpkin and the cranberry mixture in a medium bowl.
5. To the flour mixture, add the pecans and cranberry-pumpkin mixture and stir to fully incorporate.
6. Spoon the batter into the pan, and use a rubber spatula or back of a spoon to smooth the top.
7. At this point, put a rack in the bottom of a Crockpot to elevate the pan, and then put the pan on top. You can also make foil into balls and position at the bottom of the cooker.

8. Cover and cook for 2 ¾ hours on high heat. Insert a wooden toothpick to the mixture to test for doneness. It should come out clean.

9. Move the pan to a rack and let cool for about 10 minutes. Run a spatula around the inside edges to loosen the broad from the pan.

10. Place on a cooling rack and allow to cool fully. Slice and serve.

Nutritional Information per Serving: Calories 159, Carbs 21g, Fat 65g, Protein 4g

Conclusion

We have come to the end of the book. Thank you for reading and congratulations for reading until the end.

All the recipes given here will assist you further in following the program. You can still eat delicious food while losing weight; it does not have to mean eating tasteless and unfulfilling food. Such approaches will only make you give up on your weight loss goal faster. So go slow and steady with Weight Watchers and see the results.

If you found the book valuable, can you recommend it to others? One way to do that is to post a review on Amazon.

Thank you and good luck!

P Simon

Made in the USA
Middletown, DE
07 November 2018